*To the memory
of my predecessors
Alessandro Vallebona
and Luigi Oliva*

Springer
Milano
Berlin
Heidelberg
New York
Barcelona
Budapest
Hong Kong
London
Paris
Santa Clara
Singapore
Tokyo

Double contrast barium enema

The Genoa approach

Giorgio Cittadini

Foreword by Alexander R. Margulis

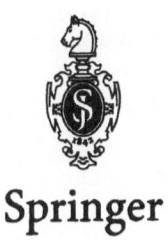

Springer

GIORGIO CITTADINI, M.D.
Professor and Chairman
Department of Radiology
University of Genoa School of Medicine
San Martino Hospital, Genoa, Italy

CONTRIBUTORS

NICOLA PANDOLFO, M.D.
Associate Professor of Surgery
University of Genoa, Italy

NOVARINO RIZZOLA, M.D.
Consultant Psychiatrist
Formerly Researcher, University of Genoa, Italy

FRANCESCO SARDANELLI, M.D.
Vice-Chief, Radiology Unit
San Martino Hospital, Genoa, Italy

GIAMPIERO TOSI, Ph.D.
Director, Physics Division
European Institute of Oncology, Milan, Italy

© Springer-Verlag Italia, Milano 1998

Softcover reprint of the hardcover 1st edition 1998

ISBN-13: 978-88-470-2219-5   e-ISBN-13: 978-88-470-2217-1
DOI: 10.1007/978-88-470-2217-1

Library of Congress Cataloging-in-Publication Data: Cittadini, Giorgio. Double contrast barium enema: the Genoa approach / Giorgio Cittadini; foreword by Alexander R. Margulis. p. cm. Includes bibliographical references. ISBN 8847000033 (hardcover) 1. Intestine, Large--Radiography. 2. Barium enema. I. Title. RC804.R6C58 1997 616.3'407572--dc21 97-40608 CIP

Typesetting: Photo Life (Milan)
Printing and binding: Staroffset (Cernusco sul Naviglio, Milan)
Cover design: Simona Colombo

SPIN: 10647820

Foreword

Carcinoma of the colon remains the second most common deadly malignant tumor afflicting humanity. It has also been shown that the great majority of colonic cancers start as polyps. It is proven, furthermore, that as with carcinoma of the breast, survival of patients found to have carcinoma of the colon is directly related to early detection. With the increasing awareness throughout the industrialized world that health care expenditures need to be carefully monitored, designing an affordable diagnostic screening approach is essential, as it is apparent that colonoscopy is too costly and too involved.

This book, by Professor Giorgio Cittadini, presents a superb approach to the performance of the double-contrast barium enema (DCBE) examination of the colon. It discusses, in great detail, the reasons for using this (the Genoa) technique, the indications for performing the double-contrast BE versus the single-contrast examination, the steps necessary to obtain a clean colon and the optimal barium sulfate suspensions to be employed.

The book deals succinctly with the BE examination in children and frankly discusses the relative merits of colonoscopy versus DCBE. An intriguing and captivating chapter on the psychologic implications of barium enemas concludes this interesting book.

The illustrations, with multiple high quality radiographic examples of pathologic conditions occurring in the colon, contribute significantly to the great value of this book, and the schematic drawings clarify its messages.

The greatest advantages of Professor Cittadini's book, however, are its clarity, succinctness and objectivity. It also makes for enjoyable reading.

Alexander R. Margulis

Acknowledgements

Even the most enthusiastic person will find it difficult to sacrifice all the time required to write a scientific book, without the support of strong encouragement. Several contributions have proved essential in this regard. First of all, the Author wishes to mention the kind attention and keen interest demonstrated in the Genoa technique by Mr. Daniel R. Martin, President of E-Z-EM. His suggestion to present this technique publicly to encourage a more careful evaluation has now been adopted with the publication of this book.

In the late '70s, many people and industries contributed to the development of the Genoa technique for the double-contrast examination of the colon. Some of them, with their determination, gave an active support to the book *Double-Contrast Barium Enema: Methodological and Technical Problems* (Verona: Cortina, 1981), which first codified the technique and led to this more comprehensive book. The Author wishes to thank Mr. John Bowman, whose assistance has been beneficial during the initial steps of the Genoa technique, especially in the development of a suitable barium suspension; Gian Andrea Rollandi, MD, researcher at the Department of Radiology, University of Genoa, and Giacomo Perelli, MD, Chief of the Radiology Unit, Hospital of Sanremo, whose contribution to the quick evolution of the technique has been crucial; Imation Italy, Milan, for the firm support provided to the research of ever more advanced screen/film radiographic systems.

A valuable strategic help has been given by our residents in Radiology Michele Bertolotto, Marco Falchi, Ilan Rosenberg and Maura Valle throughout the time required to write this book. Our radiology technician Luciano Moggia offered unlimited collaboration in order to obtain hardcopies of the radiographic images with the highest quality. Antonio Cittadini has once again offered his valuable spontaneous help in preparing all the schematic drawings presented in this book.

Eighteen Refresher Courses have been held in Genoa on the DCBE examination since 1979. None of them could have actually succeeded in propagating the technique and promoting its growth without the constant friendly and valuable help of Dr. Michele Garlisi, Director of Bracco Diagnostic Imaging, Milan, and his collaborator, Mr. Valtero Canepa.

Genoa, May 1997   *Giorgio Cittadini*

Table of Contents

1 Si parva licet componere magnis...

A fifteen-year dispute has been going on between double-contrast (DC) and single-contrast (SC) barium enema (BE) supporters [1-22]. It has been by now demonstrated that DCBE, for its greater anatomic resolution, is a more sensitive method to identify early inflammatory processes, polyps with less than one centimeter diameter (with respect to which clinical management is modernly becoming more aggressive [23]) as well as small carcinomas. Hence, this method has played an ever more important role in the radiographic examination of the colon.

This was also confirmed by the results of a second survey conducted by Thoeni and Margulis [24] ten years after the previous one, according to which "the use of double-contrast technique has markedly increased in 175 leading centers in the world... and it appears to be the primary method of examination in 56% of the centers polled".

In our department, for what concerns the present status of the radiographic examination of the colon, the opinion of Margulis and Thoeni [25] is commonly shared:

- SCBE is the method of choice for the very young, the very old, the seriously ill, and the very disabled patient, and it should be used for suspected obstruction and fistulization;
- DCBE should be employed in any patient with repeated guaiac-positive stool, in patients with family history of polyps and/or cancer, in patients with follow-up studies for polyp and/or cancer, in inflammatory bowel disease, and in the search for unknown cause of anemia and weight loss;
- the biphasic examination, that is the extemporary combination of SCBE and DCBE, should

be used in all patients with incomplete or equivocal examination by one of the two methods, or in patients with severe diverticulosis and questionable polyps.

There is a growing opinion that these studies are complementary, each possessing advantages in different clinical sets [26], and in the presence of diverticulosis a combination of single- and double-contrast techniques can significantly improve the sensitivity of the examination in the detection of polypoid lesions [14].

Why, then, despite the proven advantages of DCBE, has SCBE been used for such a long time and still it is in many institutions as routine method for the radiologic examination of the colon? There are several significant reasons for this.

The first reason is *conservatism*: who is likely to abandon the known for the unknown? Young [8], in his work *The double contrast barium enema: Why bother?*, underlines some of the elements that may account for this attitude: "What was good enough yesterday is good enough today... There may also be a belief that an old dog cannot learn new tricks... These beliefs are all too often encouraged by a trickle of articles in the world literature that set out to refute the value of DCBE and thereby add fuel to the dying embers of 'conservational' radiology".

The second reason is the fact that *the techniques required for the double-contrast barium enema are demanding and "costly" for both the radiologist and the patient*.

The third reason is *the need for an exhaustive analysis of the new radiographic signs*, for which Laufer [27] is to be credited with his "Double contrast gastrointestinal radiology with endoscopic correlation", whereas radiologists are too much accustomed to reasoning in the conventional terms of plus and minus images.

A fourth reason may be *the realization of possible perceptive, technical, or combined, causes of error on barium enema examinations*, as reported for the first time by Ott, Gelfand and Ramquist [28] and later examined in-depth also by other Authors [9, 29-31].

The need to have concurrent testing of SCBE and DCBE on the same patients is the fifth reason. The results obtained by De Roos, Hermans, Shaw et al. [32] on 425 patients have confirmed that DCBE is a better screening method for rectal and colon polyps.

Not to mention *the strong "restraining" effect of the timeworn debate on the role of colonoscopy* [33]: is it to be considered as a first choice examination? Or merely as an alternative? Or is it a complementary method? On this issue, refer to our comments in Chapter 21. Despite the "sectarian" pro-endoscopy opinions still maintained by many gastroenterologists [34-37], here we would just like to mention the proper comment made by Gelfand [38] when he stated that "the overall diagnostic yield of the barium enema is most likely higher than that of colonoscopy, primarily because of the inability of the latter examination to consistently visualize the entire colon".

In this context, the great amount of investigations that have progressively led to the definition of the Genoa DCBE technique (Oliva and Cittadini [39]) was aimed at propagating the use of this method. This was obtained by simplifying many relevant technical aspects – yet in full respect of colon functions – as well as by extending its application field to the detection of motor function abnormalities which characterize the so frequent irritable bowel syndrome (IBS).

Quite surprisingly, some technical aspects which were overcome more than 15 years ago by the Genoa technique are still reported in the literature as apparently original works. For example, the achievement of good intestinal cleansing in patients following a diet enriched with non-absorbable fibers [40]; the fact that cleansing enemas are no longer required [41, 42]; the good intestinal preparation obtained with a rational administration in time of cathartics; the interaction between magnesium ions and barium suspensions [43]; the fluoroscopic/radiographic technique; the fact that sophisticated radiographic imaging with high spatial resolution is not all in all necessary [44]. To all this, we have also to add the direct contribution given by radiology to the diagnosis of IBS, which is no longer obtained only through exclusion of organic diseases [45].

Has a wider propagation of the Genoa technique been hampered by the failure to present it in a more commonly mastered language? Indeed, it may be useful to remember that DCBE of the colon was apparently first performed by Hugo Laurel in Uppsala, but because his report was in Swedish, a not commonly mastered language, he was not given credit for the adoption of this method [25]. Actually we do not know whether this is to be considered as a limitation in the Author's publication, rather than a limitation in the language-biased bibliographic research by other Authors.

Anyway, this book aims to fulfill such a gap by presenting, at international level, the final version of a technique which has been thoroughly tested and proven in the field for more than 15 years since its application. In our San Martino University Hospital, Genoa, Italy, the biggest in Europe, with 4,500 beds and up to 6 independent Radiology Departments, approximately 41,500 DCBE examinations have been carried out with this technique. The results from a recently conducted survey show that 82% of Italian Centers use the intestinal preparation technique we apply in Genoa, and 63% follow the Genoa technique thoroughly.

The Genoa technique will be described in this book (Chapter 4), after a brief note on DCBE history (Chapter 2) and a description of its advantages from an anatomical viewpoint (Chapter 3). A short description of the anatomy and physiology of the large intestine is briefly given with regard to problems which may be raised by DCBE (Chapters 5 and 6). The role of diet, purgatives and cleansing enema are described in Chapters 7-9. The core of the Genoa technique – the simple, innocuous and effective method for cleansing the large bowel without enemas – is fully discussed in Chapter 10. Finally, pharmaceutical issues are discussed (Chapters 11-13), together with radiological (Chapters 14-16), X-ray protection (Chapter 17), clinical (Chapters 18-21) and psychological aspects (Chapter 22) which have led to the development of the currently employed technique. In other words, the whys and the wherefores of the Genoa technique.

Si parva licet componere magnis (i.e. if we were to

compare small things with big things), we would like to compare our situation with what happened to the Malmö technique, which was officially presented in a book by Welin and Welin [46] after 17 years of field practice.

Despite the detachment by which a scientific book should be presented, we cannot deny that we are anxious about the acceptance of this book. Constructive criticisms will be used to correct defects and further improve the qualities of the technique. Though many Authors take an extremely conservative attitude towards any changes to a personally developed technique, to believe that improvements are impossible would be an act of conceitedness and would mean to ignore the *vis in pectore* of valuable scientific research.

References

1. Laufer I (1976) The double-contrast enema: myths and misconceptions. Gastrointest Radiol 1:19-31
2. Miller RE, Lehman G (1976) The barium enema. Is it obsolete? JAMA 235:2842-2844
3. Margulis AR (1976) Is the double-contrast examination of the colon the only acceptable radiographic examination? Radiology 119:741-742
4. Shirakabe H, Kumakura K, Nishizawa M et al (1959) Method of X-ray examination and limits of diagnosis of the large intestine. Jpn J Clin Med 17:1729-1745
5. Maruyama M (1978) Radiologic diagnosis of polyps and carcinoma of the large bowel. Tokyo
6. Evers K, Laufer I, Gordon RL et al (1981) Double-contrast enema examination for detection of rectal carcinoma. Radiology 140:635-639
7. Gelfand DW, Ott DJ (1981) Single- vs. double-contrast gastrointestinal studies: Critical analysis of reported statistics. AJR 137:523-528
8. Young J (1982) The double contrast barium enema: Why bother? South Med J 75:46-55
9. Kelvin FM (1982) Radiologic approach to the detection of colorectal neoplasia. Radiol Clin North Am 20:743-759
10. Klaude JV, Harty RF. Sensitivity of single contrast barium enema with regard to colorectal disease as diagnosed by colonoscopy. Eur J Radiol 1982; 2:290-292
11. Johnson CD, Carlson HC, Taylor WF et al (1983) Barium enemas of carcinoma of the colon: Sensitivity of double- and single-contrast studies. AJR 140:1143-1149
12. Czembirek H, Sommer G, Wittich G et al (1983) Ergebnisse der kolon-doppelkontrast-untersuchungen. Radiologe 23:304-311
13. Beggs I, Thomas BM (1983) Diagnosis of carcinoma of the colon by barium enema. Clin Radiol 34:423-425
14. De Roos A, Hermans J, Op den Orth JO (1984) Polypoid lesions of the sigmoid colon: A comparison of single-contrast, double-contrast, and biphasic examinations. Radiology 151:597-599
15. Ott DJ, Chen YM, Gelfand DW et al (1986) Single-contrast vs. double-contrast barium enema in the detection of colonic polyps. AJR 146:993-996
16. Rex DK, Lehman GA, Lappas JC et al (1986) Sensitivity of double-contrast barium study for left-colon polyps. Radiology 158:69-72
17. Gelfand DW, Chen YM, Ott DJ (1987) Detection of colonic polyps on single-contrast barium studies: emphasis on the elderly. Radiology 164:333-337
18. Ott DJ, Scharling ES, Chen YM et al (1989) Barium enema examination: Sensitivity in detecting colonic polyps and carcinomas. South Med J 82:197-200
19. Ott DJ, Scharling ES, Chen YM et al (1989) Positive predictive value and post-test probability of diagnosis of colonic polyp on single- and double-contrast barium enema. AJR 153:735-739
20. Kerner SP (1989) Single-contrast versus double-contrast barium enema. Appl Radiol 18:26-30
21. Nakano H, Jaramillo E, Watanabe M et al (1992) Intestinal tuberculosis: Findings on double-contrast barium enema. Gastrointest Radiol 17:108-114
22. Freedman SN (1992) The role of barium enema in detecting colorectal disease: A radiologist's perspective. Postgrad Med 92:245-251
23. Feczko PJ, Bernstein MA, Halpert RD et al (1984) Small colonic polyps: A reappraisal of their significance. Radiology 152:301-303
24. Thoeni RF, Margulis AR (1988) The state of radiographic technique in the examination of the colon. Radiology 167:7-12
25. Margulis AR, Thoeni RF (1988) The present status of the radiologic examination of the colon. Radiology 167:1-5
26. Demas BE, Margulis AR (1984) Combined use of double- and single-contrast barium enema in the evaluation of suspected colonic disease. Gastrointest Radiol 9:241-245
27. Laufer I (1979) Double contrast gastrointestinal radiology with endoscopic correlation. Philadelphia, Saunders
28. Ott DJ, Gelfand DW, Ramquist NA (1980) Causes of error in gastrointestinal radiology. II. Barium enema examination. Gastrointest Radiol 5:99-105
29. Kelvin FM, Gardiner R, Vas W et al (1981) Colorectal carcinoma missed on double contrast barium enema study: a problem in perception. AJR 137:307-313
30. Markus JB, Somers S, O'Malley BP et al (1990) Double-contrast barium enema studies: Effect of multiple reading on perception error. Radiology 175:155-156
31. Anderson N, Cook HB, Coates R (1991) Colonoscopically detected colorectal cancer missed on barium enema. Gastrointest Radiol 16:123-127
32. De Roos A, Hermans J, Shaw PC et al (1985) Colon polyps and carcinomas: Prospective comparison of the single- and double-contrast examination in the same patients. Radiology 154:11-13
33. Stevenson GW (1990) Radiology and endoscopy: commentary. Annu Gastrointest Endosc P 11-14
34. Thorson AG, Christensen MA, Davis SJ (1986) The role of colonoscopy in the assessment of patients with colorectal cancer. Dis Colon Rectum 29:306-311
35. Van Ness MM, Chobanian SJ, Winters C Jr et al (1987) A study of patient acceptance of double-contrast barium ene-

ma and colonoscopy. Which procedure is preferred by patients? Arch Intern Med 147:2175-2176

36. Hixson LJ, Sampliner RE, Chernin M et al (1989) Limitation of combined flexible sigmoidoscopy and double contrast barium enema in patients with rectal bleeding. Eur J Radiol 9:254-257

37. Norfleet RG, Ryan ME, Wyman JB et al (1991) Barium enema versus colonoscopy for patients with polyps found during flexible sigmoidoscopy. Gastrointest Endosc 37:531-534

38. Gelfand DW (1988) Gastrointestinal Radiology: A Short History and Predictions for the Future. AJR 150:727-730

39. Oliva L, Cittadini G (1981) Il clisma a doppio contrasto: problemi metodologici e tecnici. Verona: Cortina

40. Fork FT (1988) Wheat fibre before radiography of the large bowel. Acta Radiol 29:375

41. Mundinger A, Dengel H, Leibersperger H (1990) Vergleichende studie zur vorbereitung der doppelkontrastuntersuchung des kolons: Prepacol versus rizinuskapseln mit reinigungseinlauf. Radiologe 30:34-38

42. Chakraverty S, Hughes T, Keir J et al (1994) Preparation of the colon for double-contrast barium enema: Comparison of Picolax, Picolax with cleansing enema and Citramag (2 sachets) – A randomized prospective trial. Clin Radiol 49:566-569

43. Conry BG, Jones S, Bartram CI (1987) The effect of oral magnesium-containing bowel preparation agents on mucosal coating by barium sulphate suspensions. Br J Radiol 60:1215-1219

44. Kastan DJ, Ackerman LV, Feczko PJ (1987) Digital gastrointestinal imaging: The effect of pixel size on detection of subtle mucosal abnormalities. Radiology 162:853-856

45. Ritsema GH, Thijn CJP (1991) Painful irritable bowel syndrome and sigmoid contractions. Clin Radiol 43:113-116

46. Welin S, Welin G (1976) The double contrast examination of the colon. Experience with the Welin modification. Stuttgart: Thieme

2 A short long history

Since the very beginning, DCBE has had a difficult life. When, in 1923, the German surgeon Fischer [1] had the idea of associating barium and air to study rectal tumors, thus attempting for the first time the double contrast examination of the colon, times were not yet ready for such a breakthrough. A still totally insufficient intestinal cleansing (so that fecal residues would often be interpreted as organic lesions), the lack of barium suspensions with sufficient mucosal adhesiveness (the attempt was also made in those days of replacing barium with thorium dioxide!), technical limits of radiographic recording systems, would all seriously affect the outcome. The attempt made by Weber [2] to develop a more refined, yet unfortunately difficult to implement DCBE technique, was also a failure.

Hence, this method was abandoned for a long time, in favor of other methods which would better suit the technology and know-how available at that time:

- the study of mucosal relief after barium evacuation, which had convinced supporters (Robinson [3], and, more recently, Marshak and Lindner [4]);
- the Gianturco technique [5], which associates a low concentration barium suspension with high kilovoltage radiography, thus obtaining a kind of semi-transparent enema.

With the Gianturco technique, also relatively small lesions projecting into the colon lumen can be detected by transparency, being demonstrated by filling defects revealed in the slightly radiopaque barium-filled colon. The effectiveness of this technique is confirmed by the amount of detected polyps in adults: 2.7% (Gianturco and Miller [6]).

This was more or less the situation when Welin [7-9], after a massive study which lasted 18 years (1953-1970), recognized that a whole series of essential requirements were to be met before DCBE could actually express its full resolution potential. Namely:

- perfect intestinal cleansing;
- availability of effective antisecretory and hypotonic drugs;
- availability of suitable barium suspensions to form a thin and homogeneous film adherent to the colon mucosa;
- radiographic technique standardization, to rapidly obtain a series of reference radiographs.

With his technique, Welin could detect polyps in 12.4% of patients, which is the same figure given by the autopsy findings of Malmö pathologists. In this context, the really fundamental element is the achievement of a perfect intestinal cleansing, for which tannic acid is largely employed both in cleansing enemas as well as in the barium suspension. Tannic acid, by irritating the colon mucosa, stimulates contractions throughout the colon thus leading to a thorough expulsion of gases and feces. Also, through its astringent action and inhibition of mucosal secretion and oozing of fluids into the colon lumen, it facilitates adhesion of barium sulfate onto the mucosa.

However, following a few lethal accidents, especially among children, probably due to overdosage and secondary to intestinal perforation and some degree of liver toxicity [10,11], in 1964 the United States Food and Drug Administration banned the use of tannic acid for cleansing enemas in humans. Alternative solutions were not easily found and only in 1970 were substances like cascara sagrada and magnesium sulfate proposed for oral administration to clean the large bowel [12]. This solution was still in use in 1972, when tannic acid was reintroduced in clinical practice, but with restrictions on the amount allowed.

The parsimonious use of cleansing enemas in the Welin technique, which are mainly employed where torpid intestinal activity is to be expected, is indeed a significant technical progress, since patients as well as medical staff are released from a procedure of difficult execution, poorly accepted from a psychological point of view and not without drawbacks.

The adoption in 1961 of the hyperhydration scheme by Brown [13] is a further step forward. With hyperhydration, the secondary clinical effects caused by water/salt losses due to the cathartic treatment are offset. It also prevents the colon from subtracting fluids from the barium suspension which therefore keeps unaltered its physicochemical properties.

Drugs inducing colon hypotonia, the use of barium suspensions with high mucosal adhesiveness, proper gaseous distention of the colon as well as fine radiographic techniques capable of achieving a good resolution have all progressively paved the way to a new situation in radiological colon examinations: the pathologic lesion, which is no longer viewed as filling defect or plus image, gets a more faithful representation which is much closer to its real anatomic appearance.

The post-Welin era is mainly characterized by several attempts at making the technical procedure simpler, which is a fundamental condition for its propagation. Several Authors have given their valuable contributions, among them Bret [14] and Weissman [15] in France; Altaras [16] in Germany with his "colon status" proposal; Shirakabe [17] and Maruyama [18] in Japan; Miller in the United States, with his many technical innovations [19-21]; Laufer [22], who is to be credited for the first exhaustive analysis of the principles of double contrast diagnosis; Gelfand [23] for his careful review on the importance of an accurate intestinal preparation.

In Italy, along with the Altaras technique, which is still largely employed, the so-called Genoa technique has developed [24-27]. As mentioned above, it aims at simplifying and at the same time, standardizing DCBE implementation, so that each step in the procedure becomes an objective act independent of any off-hand decision which may be taken by the operator (with the obvious exception of those cases where the procedure needs to be modified for diagnostic reasons or because of the patient conditions). In other words, the Genoa technique is designed as a ready-made suit, for which adaptations are only occasionally required, rather than a suit tailor-made to each individual patient. All this, with the obvious advantage of faster execution.

The technique features are the following:

- intestinal preparation of the patient obtained – without cleansing enemas – through the properly sequenced association of cathartics, by which motor activation of the colon precedes that of the small intestine, and hyperhydration;
- the use of a low density and low viscosity barium suspension administered "by gravity", which interacts with magnesium ions left in the colon lumen from the previous phase;
- large bowel hypotonia induced by anticholinergic drugs without deleting any signs of functional colonopathy (IBS);
- limited use of fluoroscopy, which is the major irradiation source for the patient;
- rigorous sequence of radiographic documentation aiming at simplifying the work of the X-ray technician.

Today radiologists are daily confronted by endoscopists. Like the latter ones, radiologists can examine the mucosa surface of the colon, with greater practical limitations yet with the advantage of higher simplicity and a more complete and panoramic view of the large bowel. It is commonly admitted that the number of colonoscopies for diagnostic reasons decreases proportionally to the radiologist's skills and reliability.

Modern procedures for the study of colon and rectal walls – US, CT and MRI – have not made indications to DCBE less valuable. Indeed, DCBE today, at a time of its full technical and interpretation maturity, is more than ever a technique offering great diagnostic accuracy and still capable of playing a major role in the imaging study of the large bowel [28-30].

In fact, in some countries, like in Italy for example, where endoscopy is largely available and techniques to study the colon wall are very much employed, the number of barium enema investigations of the colon have been only moderately reduced since 1987 [31]. The intense work of propagation among radiologists of simple, rapid and effective DCBE techniques may have contributed to this.

References

1. Fischer AW (1923) Über eine neue röntgenologische Untersuchungsmethode des Dickdarms: Kombination von Kontrasteinlauf und Luftaufblähung. Klin Wochenschr 2:1595-1598

2. Weber HM (1931) Roentgenologic demonstration of polypoid lesions and polyposis of large intestine. AJR 25:577-589

3. Robinson JM (1954) Detection of small lesions of the large bowel; barium enema versus double contrast. Calif Med 81:321-324

4. Marshak RH, Lindner AE (1970) The radiology corner. Am J Gastroenterol 53:478-481

5. Gianturco C (1950) High-voltage technic in the diagnosis of polypoid growths of the colon. Radiology 55:27-29

6. Gianturco C, Miller G (1953) Routine search for colonic polyps by high voltage radiography. Radiology 60:496-499

7. Welin S (1958) Modern trends in diagnostic roentgenology of the colon. Br J Radiol 31:453-464

8. Welin S (1967) Results of the Malmo technique of the colon examination. JAMA 199:369-371

9. Welin S, Welin G (1976) The double contrast examination of the colon. Experience with the Welin modification. Stuttgart: Thieme

10. Mc Alister WH, Anderson MS, Bloomberg GR, Margulis AR (1963) Lethal effects of tannic acid in barium enema. Radiology 80:756-773

11. Luke HH, Hodge KE, Patt JL (1963) Fatal liver damage after barium enemas containing 1% tannic acid. Can Med Assoc J 89:1111-1114

12. Welin S (1971) Examination and cleansing of the large bowel. J Belge Radiol 54:1-6

13. Brown GR (1961) A new approach to colon preparation for barium enema: Preliminary report. Univ Mich Med Bull 27:225-230

14. Bret P, Piante M (1972) Radiologie colique en double contraste. Technique de routine. Ann Radiol 15:637-644

15. Weissman A, Clot M, Grellet J (1978) Réalisation pratique du double contrast colique. J Radiol Electrol Med Nucl 59: 299-302

16. Altaras J (1982) Radiologischer Atlas, Kolon und Rektum. München: Urban & Schwarzenberg

17. Shirakabe H, Kumakura K, Nishizawa M et al (1959) Method of X-ray examination and limits of diagnosis of the large intestine. Nippon Rinsho (Jpn J Clin Med) 17:1729-1745

18. Maruyama M (1978) Radiologic diagnosis of polyps and carcinoma of the large bowel. Tokyo: Igaku-Shoin

19. Miller RE (1964) Barium enema examination with large-bore tubing and drainage. Radiology 82:905-911

20. Miller RE (1969) A new enema tip. Radiology 92:1492

21. Miller RE (1970) Simple apparatus for decubitus films with horizontal beam. Radiology 97:682-688

22. Laufer I (1979) Double contrast gastrointestinal radiology with endoscopic correlation. Philadelphia: Saunders

23. Gelfand DW, Chen MYM, Ott DJ (1991) Preparing the colon for the barium enema examination. Radiology 178: 609-613

24. Cittadini G., Perelli G, Santolini ME (1977) Tecnica di realizzazione del clisma a doppio contrasto. Il Radiologo 16/2:31-36

25. Cittadini G, Rollandi GA, Giribaldi M (1980) Su un metodo semplice innocuo ed efficiente di pulizia intestinale senza clisteri. Radiol Med 66:415-420

26. Oliva L, Cittadini G (1981) Il clisma a doppio contrasto: problemi metodologici e tecnici. Verona: Cortina

27. Cittadini G, Rollandi GA, Russo S (1986) Intestino crasso. In: Cittadini G, Tecnica di studio a doppio contrasto del tubo digerente: la via italiana. Genova: Ecig, pp. 89-110

28. Laufer I (1994) Current status of barium studies of the gastrointestinal tract. Proceedings ECR '94, Singapore

29. Reeders JWAJ, Bakker ADJ, Rosenbusch G (1994) Contemporary radiological examination of the lower gastrointestinal tract. In: Tytgat GNJ, Reeders JWAJ Diagnostic Imaging of the Gastrointestinal Tract, Part I, London: Baillière Tindall

30. Reeders JWAJ, Rosenbusch G (1994) Clinical Radiology and Endoscopy of the Colon. New York: Thieme

31. Cittadini G (1994) Radiologia gastrointestinale – Un crocevia pericoloso: ecoendoscopia o endoecografia? Il Radiologo 33/2:92-94

3 Why double contrast barium enema?

In 1976 an article by Margulis [1] published in the "Opinion" column of *Radiology* was entitled: "Is the double contrast examination of the colon the only acceptable radiographic examination?". In this article the Author also asks the following question: "Does this mean that radiologists not performing a double-contrast examination as the only radiographic procedure are wrong?".

Today it is possible to reply to this question in quantitative terms, based on a significant amount of experimental data which almost exclusively concern polyps and carcinomas, because of the clinical importance of an early diagnosis of these lesions which remain asymptomatic for a long time (Fig. 1). However, also qualitative considerations on the anatomic resolution become important to settle the timeworn debate already mentioned in Chapter 1 between SCBE and DCBE supporters.

The frequency of polyps seen in different radiological reports ranges from 1% to 7.8% for the SCBE, from 9.8% to 13.1% for the DCBE [2]. The latter figures compare favorably with the average autopsy incidence (12.4%) of colon polyps. SCBE and DCBE seem to be equally sensitive in detecting colon cancer above the proctoscopic level, with an error rate of 4.8% and 4.7%, respectively [3].

In the first of two important reports by Ott, Scharling, Chen et al. [4], the sensitivity of SCBE and DCBE in detecting colonic polyps and carcinomas is 82% and 91%, respectively. For lesions 1 cm or more in size the sensitivity is similar (91% vs. 95%), but for smaller polyps it is fairly different (70% vs. 88%). In other words, there is little difference in the overall sensitivity between SCBE and

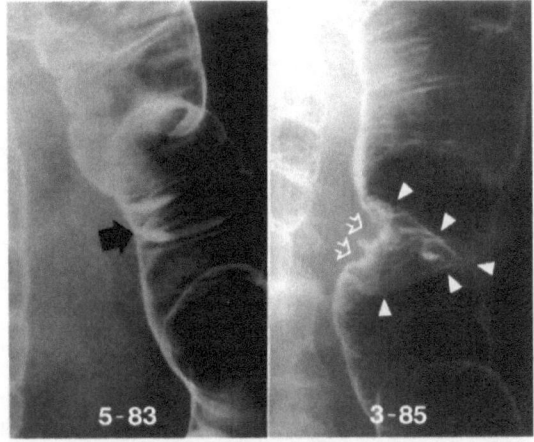

Fig. 1. Polyp/carcinoma sequence. The sessile polyp lesion (*arrow*), occasionally identified in May 1983, was considered by the physician to be sufficiently small (7 mm) to justify a watchful waiting. In March 1985, the appearance of occult blood in the feces led to a control examination. The lesion had grown along the adjacent semilunar fold infiltrating it thoroughly (*arrowheads*). The basal indentation (*open arrow*) is per se indication of transformation to invasive carcinoma

DCBE for the detection of large polyps and carcinomas, but DCBE is more sensitive than SCBE for detecting polyps smaller than 1 cm. In the second report [5], the positive predictive value for colonic polyps on the SCBE was 82% (79% for 5- to 10-mm polyps) compared with 92% for DCBE (94% for 5- to 10-mm polyps).

SCBE and DCBE were compared in 425 patients examined with both procedures during the same session [6]. In patients with carcinoma, there was no significant difference between the two modalities. DCBE was far superior to SCBE for detection of colonic and rectal polyps. However, the methods appeared to be complementary in the sigmoid and cecum.

Optimizing the technical features of SCBE as well as the procedure to be followed by the radiologist may indeed yield significant results. In a study based on the detection of polyps, 66% of lesions 5 to 9 mm in size, and 94% of those 10 mm or larger were detected radiographically; SCBE had a positive predictive value of 86% and a false-positive rate of 14% [7].

False-negative perception errors are a significant problem in the interpretation of DCBE studies, and multiple reading is an effective way to reduce this error [8,9]. In a report by Markus, Somers, O'Malley et al. [10], the sensitivity for a single reader was 70.2%, whereas the corresponding average double and triple reading sensitivities were 83.3% and 89% for the different types of visible lesions.

All this with regard to polyps and carcinomas. But, what about the other colonic diseases? Here, important aspects of the anatomic resolution of

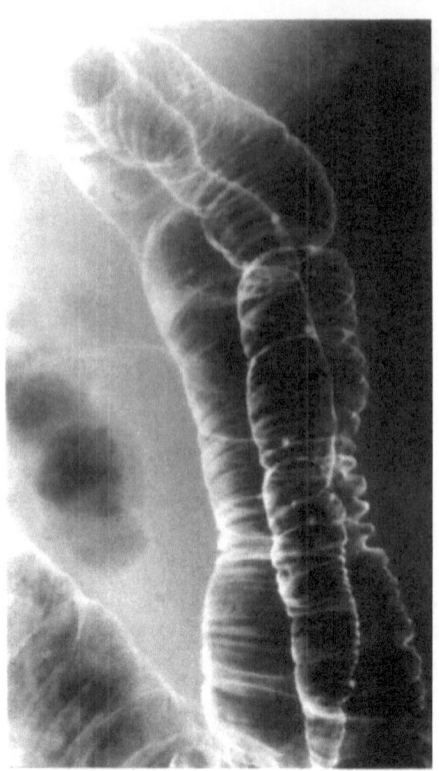

Fig. 3. The mucosal surface is widely furrowed with fine, linear and oblique reliefs giving it a coil-shaped, wool ball appearance in the left flexure. These reliefs, which are a frequent finding in patients affected by IBS, seem to be due to motor alterations of the muscularis mucosae (see also Figs. 4-6 in Chap. 19). The cock's-comb pattern along a profile portion is evidence of involvement of the circular muscular layer, thus defining a picture of IBS which is evolving towards the prediverticular phase of diverticulosis

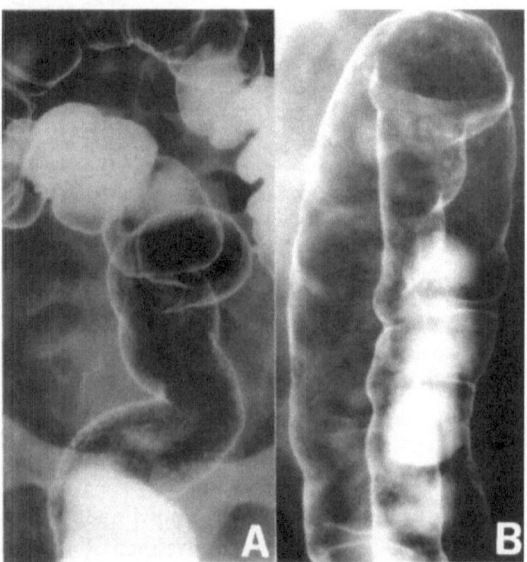

Fig. 2. With the fine analysis of mucosal surface made possible with DCBE, the granular appearance of mucosal erosions in IUC (**A**) can be properly detected. It involves the whole rectum up to the descending segment of the sigmoid. In (**B**), aphthoid ulcers typical of Crohn's disease are shown along the descending and transverse colon

the two examinations should be taken into account, rather than sensitivity. The double-contrast technique is optimal for the study of the mucosal surface and for the depiction of fine erosions and ulcers (Fig. 2). The valuable results obtained from DCBE in the detection of the initial stages of IUC and Crohn's disease have been known for a long time [11-13]. More recently, interesting data were obtained for colonic tuberculosis [14]. SCBE detects only functional phenomena, such as spasm and hypermotility of the ileocecal region; conversely, DCBE enables the direct detection of shallow ulcers with their characteristically elevated, frequently slim and transversally oriented margins.

With regard to IBS, while SCBE detects only indirect functional phenomena, such as strong circular contractions of the sigmoid colon [15], according to our experience direct signs can be detected with DCBE (Fig. 3). We shall discuss this important topic in Chapter 19.

As to the detection of the prediverticular phase of diverticulosis, DCBE gives full confidence (Fig. 4). A simple adjunct to the double-contrast technique, the sigmoid flush with low density barium, seems to improve visualization of the diverticular sigmoid and increase interpretation confidence [16].

In his Annual Oration 1989 "Bring out your barium", Simpkins [17] says that "on the basis of safety, completeness and reasonable accuracy, there is a strong case for DCBE to continue to be the initial investigation for the majority of patients with symptoms of large-bowel disease".

In our San Martino Hospital, since 1979 DCBE has been the first choice method for the radiological study of the colon; SCBE is the method of choice in some clinical situations (suspected obstruction or fistulization) and is the natural alternative in the elderly and infirm patients who cannot easily undergo a double-contrast study. In other words, priority in its implementation does not mean alleged and illogic exclusivity. The need to use the biphasic technique has in practice been felt very rarely.

We accepted this formulation of priority not only for the frequent disagreement between final assessment and radiological conclusions based in the past on SCBE – mainly in the detection of initial stages of IUC and Crohn's disease, and of small polyps and carcinomas –, but also because we thought that the higher anatomic resolution that DCBE offers, displaying the colon in a more natural and impressive form, could intrinsically be the starting point for a deeper insight into some types of pathology.

With SCBE a "mold" of the large bowel lumen is made by filling it with a radiopaque contrast medium. While plus images and stenoses appear practically always through this mold, only larger minus images – in the order of 1 cm – do show through. After evacuation, pathologic processes, though present, often fail to be seen on the radiographs (Fig. 5). Subsequent gaseous distention fails to give any reliable depiction of the mucosa unless

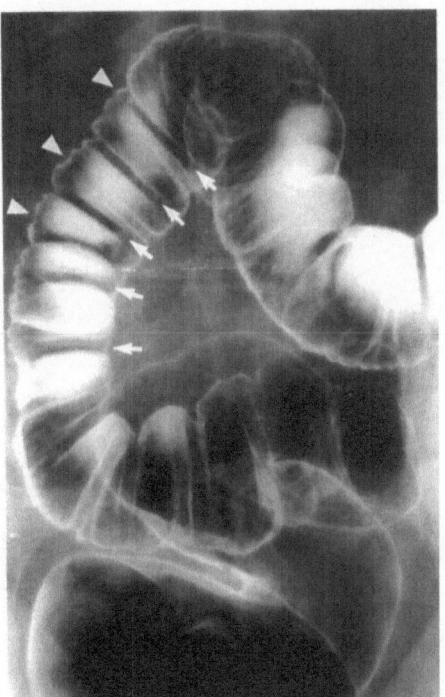

Fig. 4. Along the entire descending segment of the sigmoid, the hypertrophy of the circular muscular layer, the consequence of high pressure in this area, leads to the development of closely arranged transverse formations crossing the mucosal surface (*short arrows*). A cock's-comb like pattern is also evident along a portion of the profile (*arrowheads*). These findings are believed to be a sign of the prediverticular phase of diverticulosis

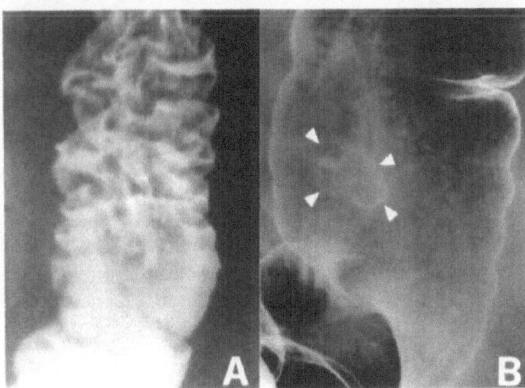

Fig. 5. SCBE and DCBE. In (**A**), in the descending-sigmoid colon detail, no sure pathologic findings could be identified with SCBE even after barium evacuation. Conversely, a polypous lesion 1.5 cm in diameter could be demonstrated with DCBE (**B**) also with a good contour definition. Histological finding: villous adenoma

it has been properly prepared, special barium suspensions are used, the radiologic technique itself is drastically modified. Yet, these last three aspects make up, in practice, the essence of DCBE.

DCBE depicts the mucosa directly by coating it with a thin layer of radiopaque contrast medium which is properly capable of adhering to it in a homogeneous and smooth way. The intestinal lumen is distended and effaced by the gaseous contrast medium. In this way, a really analytical depiction of the mucosa as well as of all pathologic formations originating from it can be achieved. Since the pathological processes of the large bowel having greatest interest for the radiologist originate from the mucosa, only with a "fine" mucosa depiction can sensitive radiographic signs, useful for diagnostic purposes, be acquired.

Interestingly enough, when the DCBE is used on a routine base, according to Bret [18], "you are likely to find what you were not looking for". Overall view (Figs. 6,7), view by transparency (Figs. 7,8), detection of protruding lesions even of a few millimeters in size (Fig. 9), fine assessment of mucosal surface (Figs. 10-12), accurate analysis of the contours (Figs. 13,14), direct demonstration of motor alterations of the muscularis mucosae and circular muscular layer (Figs. 3,4), are the features making the DCBE an extremely "resolving" examination.

Generally speaking, it can be stated that with DCBE it is possible to:

1. directly identify normal anatomic structures which by SCBE can be detected only indirectly, or which are not visible at all;

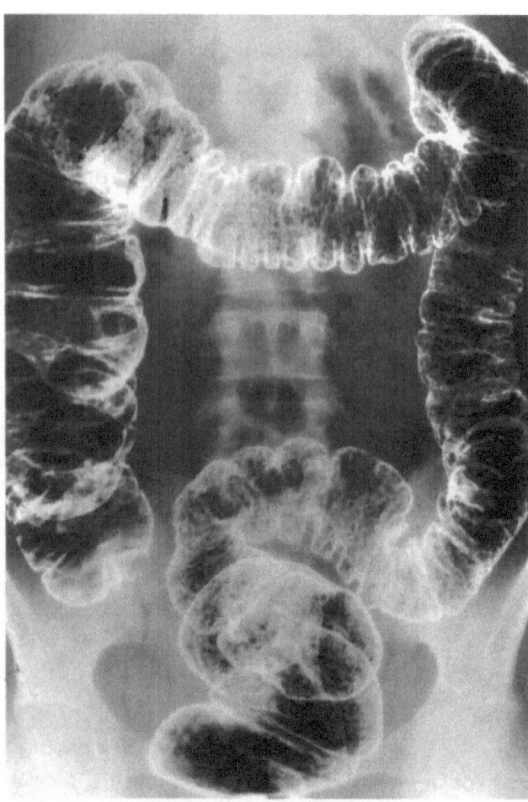

Fig. 6. Widespread familial adenomatous polyposis coli. The whole large bowel mucosal surface, from the rectum to the cecum, is carpeted with small protruding masses of a few millimeters in size, here and there more or less crowded and with a ring-like blurred contour. Considering the extent of the large bowel area involved, a total colectomy was promptly performed for the risk of carcinomatous transformation

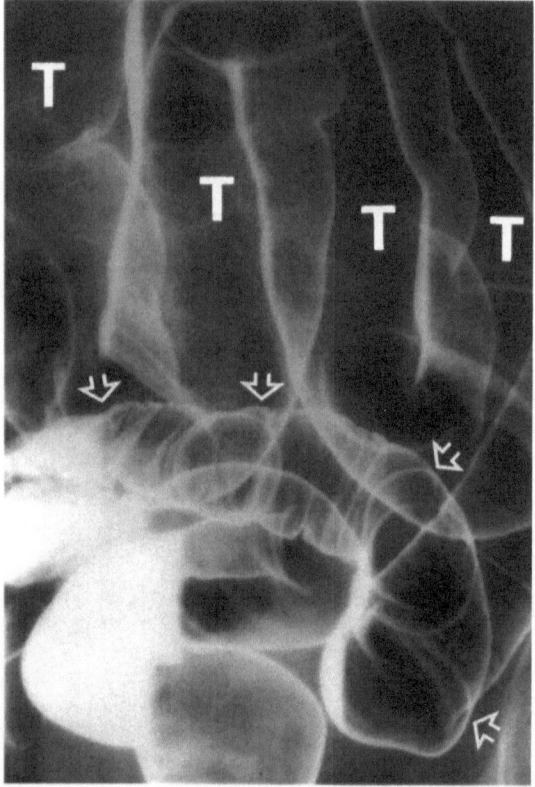

Fig. 7. The entire colonic mucosa surface can be properly analyzed even where the various segments are significantly overlapping. It should be noted that despite the conspicuously visible transverse dolichocolon taking up most of the picture (T), early prediverticular alterations of the posterior segment of the sigmoid can still be seen by transparency (*open arrows*)

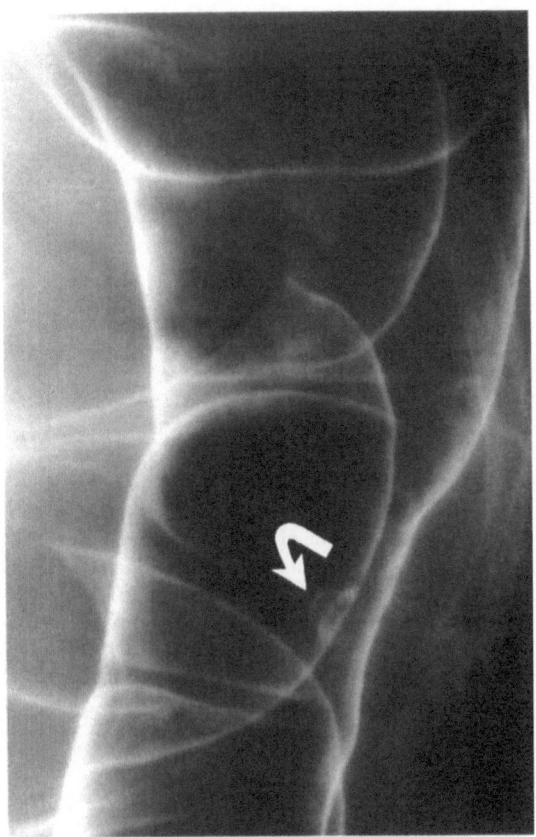

Fig. 8. This occasional sessile polyp finding (*arrow*), which is well visible by transparency within some overlapping colonic loops, takes the characteristic bowler hat appearance with inward facing apex. Site location is not possible from this image alone. As demonstrated in Fig. 1, in this type of lesion the evolution potential to invasive carcinoma should always be kept in mind

2. obtain a better definition of pathologic findings that can be assessed also by SCBE;
3. identify pathologic findings which would otherwise fail to be detected.

Normal anatomic structures

The direct and constant depiction of mucosal surface and semilunar folds (see Fig. 12 in Chap. 5) is not only interesting from a merely esthetic point of view, but it also has a significant practical interest since pathologic conditions which were undetectable for the radiologist are now visible (Figs. 4-6 in Chap. 19).

The depiction of the Bahuino's valve (Fig. 6 in Chap. 5), as well as of the terminal ileum, is almost constant, provided that proper technical maneuvers are accomplished (see Chapter 4).

The depiction of Houston and Kohlrausch's folds in the rectal ampulla (see Fig. 3 in Chap. 5) is constant. Their careful inspection is important to

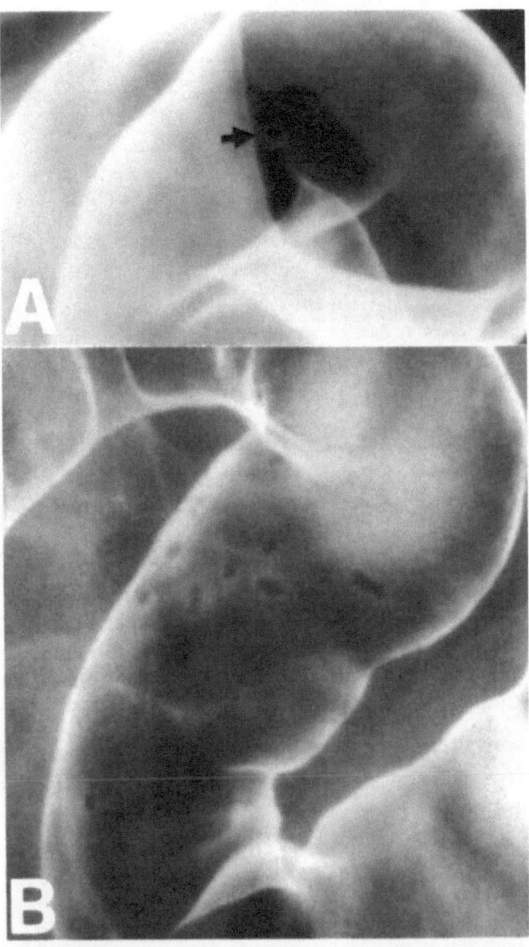

Fig. 9. Thanks to the high DCBE anatomic resolution, even very small protruding lesions can be detected. In (**A**), showing a detail of the left flexure of the colon, the mucosal coating is interrupted by a small, ball-shaped protruding mass (*arrow*) of approximately 2 mm in diameter. Since the base of the small mass forms an acute dihedral angle with the mucosa, the barium is allowed to penetrate all around the base: the X-ray full-ring rendering thus obtained, which becomes indistinct on the outside, is well visible also on print reproduction. This appearance is a sure sign of a small sessile polyp (a hyperplastic polyp in this case). In (**B**), showing a detail of the sigmoid ascending segment, small post-colitis granulomas (confirmed by the histological examination) are shown, some of them in twin formations, with sizes ranging from 1.5 to 2 mm

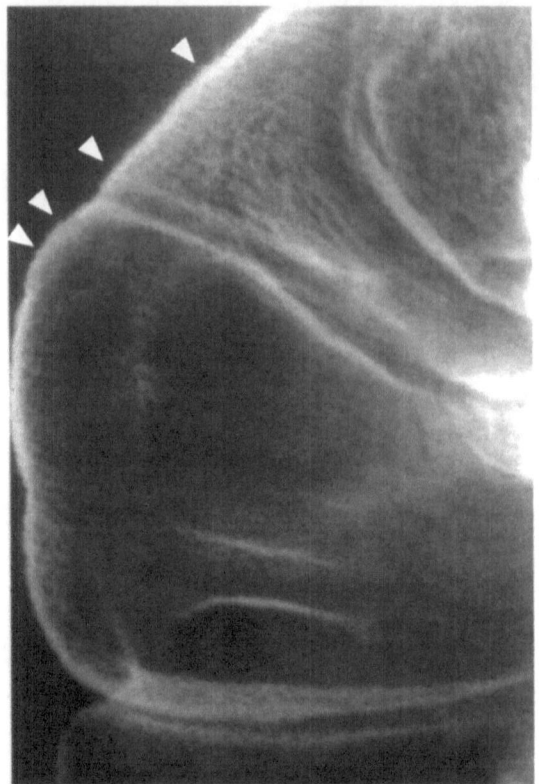

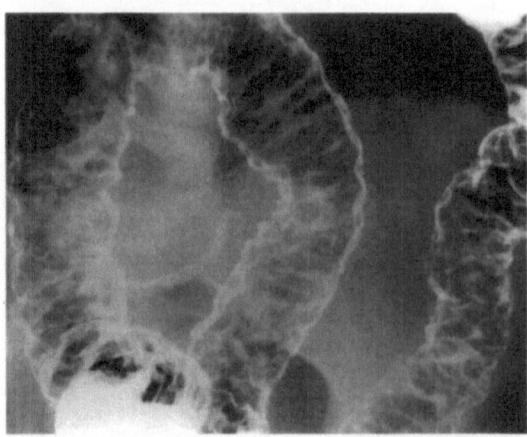

Fig. 12. Unlike small hyperplastic and adenomatous polyps, submucosal lesions raise the mucosa forming obtuse dihedral angles. No clear ring around the polyp formation can be seen at X-ray. In **(A)** (simple lymphoid hyperplasia), great care is required to spot mucosal coating alterations; in **(B)** (lymphocytic lymphoma) and in **(C)** (Hodgkin's disease) the identification of mucosal alterations is easier due to the widespread cribrate appearance of the involved segments. Infiltration of Houston fold can be observed in **(B)** (*arrowheads*)

Fig. 10. The innominate grooves. The mucosa of the colon portion illustrated here takes up a widespread velvety appearance with, here and there, a well perceptible reticular pattern. Along the colon contours, small cone-like reliefs can be observed (*arrowheads*). These mucosal sub-units are discussed in Chapter 5 (see also Figs. 14-15 therein)

Fig. 11. Pseudomembranous colitis. In this female patient, following a prolonged clindamycin treatment, the whole colonic mucosa is involved by multiple round-shaped plaque-like defects of the barium coating. Their contours and the central umbilication due to superficial punctuate ulceration are clearly shown by barium. Irregular, shaggy contours of the colon are well appreciated

detect the presence of rectal cancer, which at this level often has an infiltrative nature.

In the rectal ampulla below the level of the levator ani muscle, under favorable conditions, Morgagni's columns and sinuses can be observed quite well (see Fig. 4 in Chap. 5).

Finally, the depiction of the innominate grooves – real colonic mucosal subunits (see Fig. 10 and 14-15 in Chap. 5) – is very inconstant with the standard DCBE technique, probably because it heavily depends on patient's preparation, type of barium suspension and radiographic technique itself (see Chapter 5).

Pathologic findings better defined by DCBE

An example is given in Fig. 13 with related comments. As to polyps, the mere detection of the presence of the lesion is only one side of the problem. Indeed, an accurate dimensional and morphologic characterization is very important to quantify the risk of malignant transformation based on radiological data [19] (see Fig. 14).

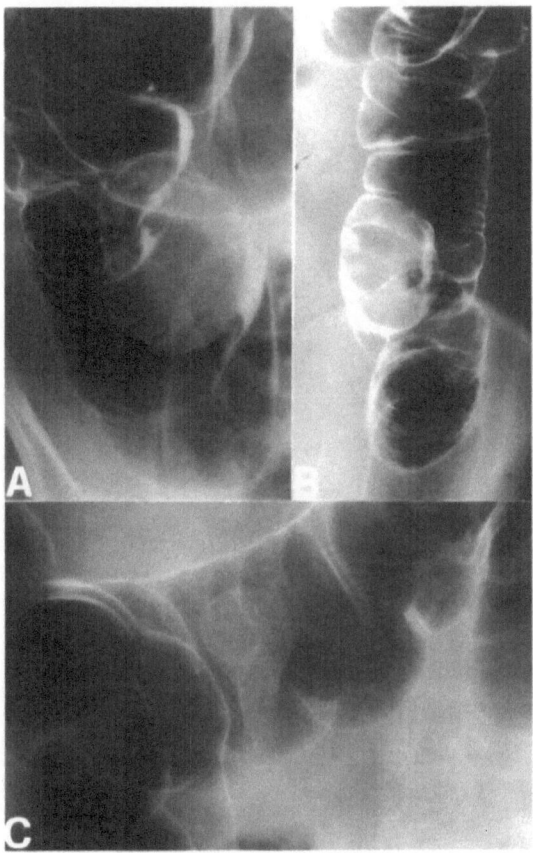

Fig. 13. The regular pattern of the three lesions (**A-C**) depicted here, which look as if drawn with calipers, can be appreciated through contour analysis, which can be done in a very accurate way with the DC examination. Despite the significant size, their somehow homogeneous transparency and no base displacement would suggest their benign nature. A sessile lipoma was diagnosed in (**A**) and pseudopedunculated lipomas in (**B**) and (**C**)

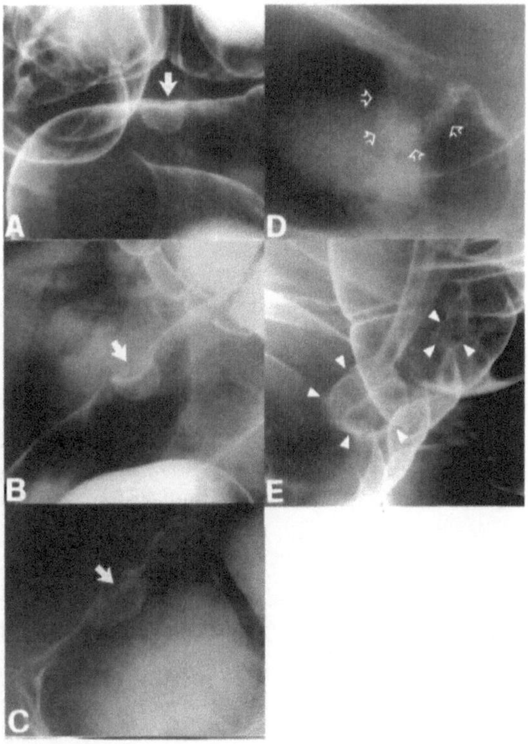

Fig. 14. Degenerated polyps. Increasing base displacement is appreciable in (**A**) and (**B**) (tubular adenomas - *arrowheads*). In (**C**) (villous adenoma), this finding is coupled with irregular surface, where the barium penetration has formed a "cauliflower" appearance. In (**D**) (tubular-villous adenoma), dual features can be identified in the large sized lesion planted in a Houston fold: the central part is smooth and regular (asterisk), while the surface is irregular and "leafy" (*hollow arrows*). In (**E**), though the peduncle seems to be regular, the heads of the two appreciable polyps (*arrowheads*) show a clearly irregular pattern, suggesting their growing nature

Pathologic findings assessable by DCBE only

Mainly, findings like lymphoid hyperplasia (see Fig. 12), the hyperemic pre-erosive phase in IUC and the aphthous ulcers of Crohn's disease (see Fig. 2), the shallow ulcers of colonic tuberculosis, small granulomatous post-colitis (Fig. 9B) and post-surgical (Fig. 15) formations, and the anastomosis appearance after colon resection (Fig. 16), are all to be included in this category.

At the end of this analysis on the reasons for our preference for DCBE, we must yet try to answer the question asked at the beginning of this chapter:

"are radiologists not performing a double-contrast examination as the only radiographic procedure wrong?". The task is simple because an answer has been given in explicit terms by the same Author Margulis together with Eisenberg in their Diamond Jubilee Lecture 1991 [20]:

"While the double-contrast technique is optimal for the study of the mucosal surface and for the depiction of aphthous ulcers and small polyps (smaller than 1 cm), a carefully performed single-contrast examination with a clean colon and adequate palpation is equally accurate for the detection of polyps 1 cm or larger. In our experience, the latter is more sensitive for detecting large neoplasms,

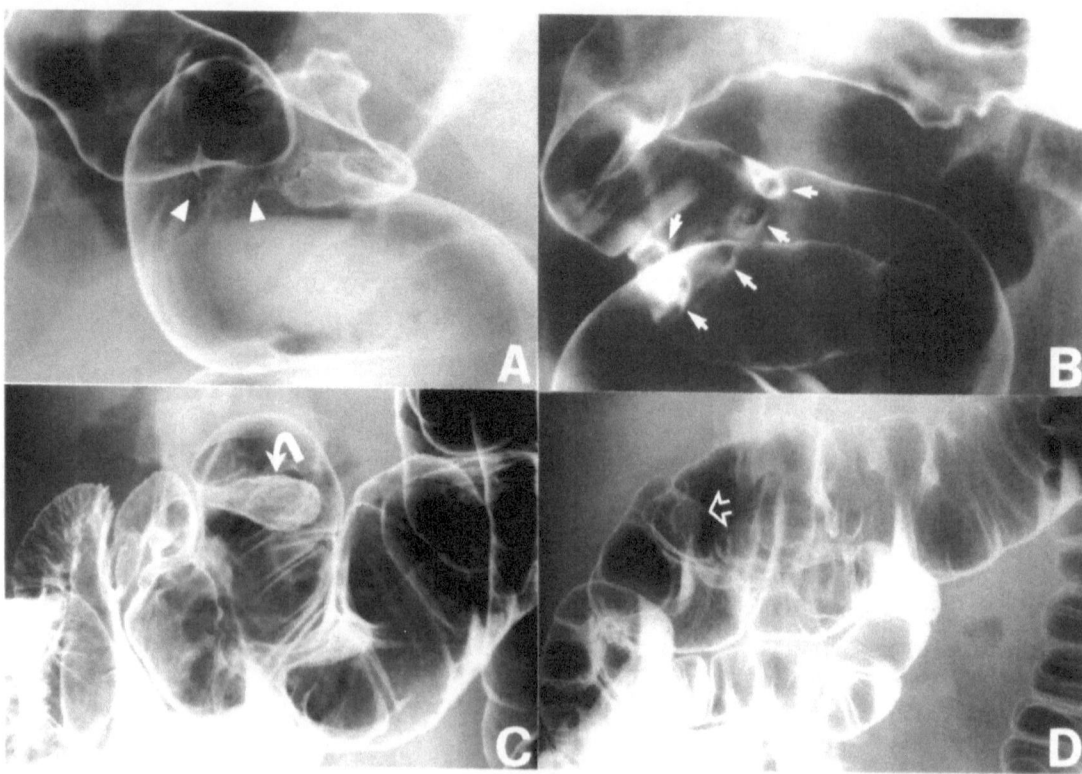

Fig. 15. Post-surgical findings. Stapled suture is well appreciable in **(A)**, looking as small interlinked rings (*arrowheads*). In **(B)**, along the sigmoid suture, which was generously oversized by the surgeon in an old patient with persistent and recurrent diverticulosis, many small granulomas have developed (*straight arrows*). In **(C)**, a few years after right hemicolectomy with side-to-side ileocolic anastomosis, a significant granulomatous development of the tobacco-box of the colonic stump is demonstrated (*curved arrow*). In **(D)**, at the level of the colonic stump (after right hemicolectomy and side-to-side ileo-transverse-anastomosis for adenocarcinoma) a small protruding recurrence with irregular margins can be observed (*open arrow*)

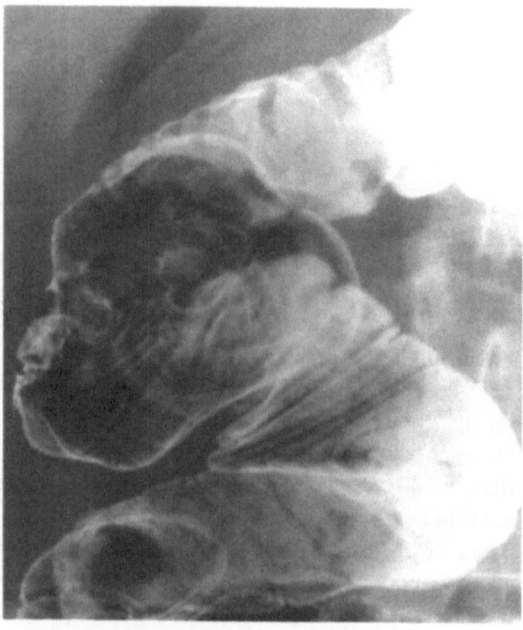

Fig. 16. The study of the anastomosis mouth and related loops becomes really analytical in a specifically targeted DCBE

sinus tracks and fistulas. The single-contrast barium enema is also the examination of choice for debilitated patients or for those who have a suspected colonic obstruction. When a double-contrast enema examination demonstrates suspicious areas, a follow-up single-contrast examination, performed after the evacuation of the air and barium introduced by the double-contrast enema, generally answers all the questions raised".

Thus the error would be to accept an exclusivity for DCBE in front of the well demonstrated important fields of action of SCBE. This means the necessity of a preliminary choice of the way to run, which, we think, is a decision that will correctly merge if clinicians and radiologists will evaluate together the best for the single patient in interdisciplinary form.

As to the radiologist, he will remember the words of Rice [21] in his 1989 oration "Lowering death rates from colorectal cancer: challenge for the 1990s":

"I am suggesting that you be as meticolous with your barium examinations as you are with your angiographic examinations and other 'special procedures'. With the opportunity to save the lives of dozens of your patients over the next decade, I do not see that there is any choice but to make this commitment".

References

1. Margulis AR (1976) Is the double-contrast examination of the colon the only acceptable radiographic examination? Radiology 119:741-742
2. Gelfand DW, Ott DJ (1981) Single- vs. double-contrast gastrointestinal studies: critical analysis of reported statistics. AJR 137:523-528
3. Johnson CD, Carlson HC, Taylor WF et al (1983) Barium enemas of carcinoma of the colon: Sensitivity of double- and single-contrast studies. AJR 140:1143-1149
4. Ott DJ, Scharling ES, Chen YM et al (1989) Barium enema examination: Sensitivity in detecting colonic polyps and carcinomas. South Med J 82:197-200
5. Ott DJ, Scharling ES, Chen YM et al (1989) Positive predictive value and post-test probability of diagnosis of colonic polyp on single- and double-contrast barium enema. AJR 153:735-739
6. De Roos A, Hermans J, Shaw PC et al (1985) Colon polyps and carcinomas: Prospective comparison of the single- and double-contrast examination in the same patients. Radiology 154:11-13
7. Gelfand DW, Chen YM, Ott DJ (1987) Detection of colonic polyps on single-contrast barium enema study: Emphasis on the elderly. Radiology 164:333-337
8. Ott DJ, Gelfand DW, Ramquist NA (1980) Causes of error in gastrointestinal radiology. II. Barium enema examination. Gastrointest Radiol 5:99-105
9. Kelvin FM, Gardiner R, Vas W et al (1981) Colorectal carcinoma missed on double contrast barium enema study: a problem in perception. AJR 137:307-313
10. Markus JB, Somers S, O'Malley BP et al (1990) Double-contrast barium enema studies: Effect of multiple reading on perception error. Radiology 175:155-156
11. Laufer I, Mullens JE, Hamilton J (1976) Correlation of endoscopy and double-contrast radiography in the early stages of ulcerative and granulomatous colitis. Radiology 118:1-5
12. Laufer I (1976) The double-contrast enema: myths and misconceptions. Gastrointest Radiol 1:19-31
13. Kelvin FM, Oddson TA, Rice RP et al (1978) Double contrast barium enema in Crohn's disease and ulcerative colitis. AJR 131:207-213
14. Nakano H, Jaramillo E, Watanabe M et al (1992) Intestinal tuberculosis: Findings on double-contrast barium enema. Gastrointest Radiol 17:108-114
15. Ritsema GH, Thijn CJP (1991) Painful irritable bowel syndrome and sigmoid contractions. Clin Radiol 43:113-116
16. Lappas JC, Maglinte DDT, Kopecky KK et al (1988) Diverticular disease: Imaging with post-double-contrast sigmoid flush. Radiology 168:35-37
17. Simpkins KC (1989) Annual Oration 1989: Bring out your barium. J Can Assoc Radiol 40:5-11
18. Bret P (1981) Radiologie de l'intestin grêle et du colon. Technique et sémiologie. Villeurbanne: Simep
19. Ushio K, Goto H, Muramatsu Y et al (1986) Significance of the profile view in the X-ray diagnosis of cancer of the digestive tract: Diagnosis of depth invasion by double contrast study. I to Cho 21:27-32
20. Margulis AR, Eisenberg RL (1991) Gastrointestinal radiology from the time of Walter B. Cannon to the 21st century. Radiology 178:297-302
21. Rice RP (1990) Lowering death rates from colorectal cancer: Challenge for the 1990s. Radiology 176:297-301

4 The Genoa technique in action

Three fundamental, sequential and interconnected phases can be distinguished in DCBE execution:

1. *intestinal preparation of the patient* (i.e. colonic lumen and mucosa preparation);
2. *double-contrast implementation* (in its two phases: uniform and thin layer barium coating of the mucosa; gaseous distention of the colonic lumen);
3. *radiographic documentation* (i.e. analytic and repeated depiction of the various colon segments on overhead radiographs and spot films, if necessary, having appropriate resolution).

In practice, every Author has some minor technical secrets for each one of these phases, thus conferring some personal features to the examination. Several actions involved in these artifices have raised perplexities among gastroenterologists and surgeons: for instance, colon cleansing obtained by repeated enemas, the use of high viscosity barium suspensions which are to be introduced pushing them forward under pressure, the large use of contact laxatives. For this reason we decided to develop a simplified and more easily acceptable technique for DCBE examination.

Some of the suggested solutions are self evident, whereas others need due consideration after a careful examination of the whys and wherefores [1]. They will be discussed in different chapters of this book. Besides, some introductory remarks are needed before describing the various sequences in the procedure to better understand the entire technique.

Intestinal preparation of the patient

In double-contrast examinations of the upper gastrointestinal tract, the implementation of the double contrast is the most delicate and complex phase. Conversely, in colon examinations, the removal of residual fecal debris is the most critical part on which the success of the whole procedure mainly depends. Our protocol for intestinal preparation is the following [2]:

1. In *standard cases*, during the three days preceding the examination the patient follows a balanced diet with medium caloric intake and with high water and low fiber content, to reduce the amount of fecal material in the colon. Written instructions are given to the patient regarding food recommended for breakfast, lunch and supper (see Tables 1 and 2 in Chap. 7). The day before the examination, the patient will skip supper. In *urgent cases*, or *when IBS is suspected*, or *when the patient has to follow a diet rich in non-absorbable fibers*, no changes are made in the diet and the next phase is immediately implemented. Besides, the results of experimental investigations have played down the importance of a preliminary diet control (see Chapter 7).

2. The day before examination, at 8:00 a.m., *156 mg of a mixture of sennosides A and B are administered orally* together with breakfast. We generally use Pursennid, Sandoz, Basel, Switzerland, named also Gentle Nature Ex-lax, 13 tablets, 12 mg each, taken in one administration, or, alternatively, X-PREP Gray Pharmaceutical (the whole bottle content diluted

with an equal amount of water). For a detailed explanation of the reason for this choice, see Chapter 10. The effect of sennosides begins 6 hours after intake through mass propulsion movements of the colon induced by direct stimulation of myoenteric plexuses as well as indirectly by inhibition of intestinal sodium reabsorption, with subsequent inflow of water by osmosis into the intestinal lumen. Since just a functional activation of the large bowel is triggered, the patient generally has two solid fecal discharges after lunch and may continue his/her normal activity as usual until early afternoon.

3. Three-four hours after lunch, when food absorption is deemed to be completed, *15 g of magnesium sulfate*, dissolved in half a glass of lukewarm water, *are administered orally*. Once in the small bowel, this hypertonic solution becomes isotonic due to the water (about 500 mL) released from the wall into the lumen. The subsequent mechanic distention induces the functional activation of the small bowel with emptying of its contents into the colon still under the effect of sennosides. Magnesium sulfate has a rapid effect by inducing the release of repeated liquid discharges which become progressively clearer during the 2-3 hours following intake.

4. A little while after intake of saline laxative, the patient will begin to drink *2 L of water or similar non carbonated beverages, over a period of 2-3 hours*. This will induce a top-bottom propulsion of colonic contents and, at the same time, forestall dehydration.

5. The patient will then *fast until examination*.

6. *No cleansing enema is required*.

This protocol of intestinal preparation, which is synthetically described in Table 1, as a rule gets a satisfying compliance out of the patient, is generally well tolerated and no more than 14% of patients spontaneously report specific complaints. If correctly performed, valid intestinal preparation is achieved in more than 90% of cases (see Chapter 10).

Great importance is to be given to timing and dosages to obtain a combined effect from cathartics to be administered in a proper sequence for colon activation, small intestine activation, top-bottom propulsion and patient hydration.

Colon hypotonization

Reduction in colon segmentation and basal tone is important for a successful double-contrast examination. For this purpose, 20 mg of hyoscine N-butylbromide (Buscopan, Boehringer Ingelheim) are administered i.v. on a routine base during the examination as soon as the emptying of surplus barium suspension in the colon lumen is completed and just before air insufflation. The drug acts on control mechanisms of the neurovegetative system on colon tone and motility by specifically inhibiting the muscarinic parasympathetic component (see Chapter 11). Owing to the mild level and transitoriety of symptomatic side-effects, such as dryness of the mouth, tachycardia and blurring vision, the drug is of easy control and use, with few absolute contraindications.

Table 1. The Genoa protocol of intestinal preparation

3 days before	
	beginning of a balanced diet with medium caloric intake and with high water and low fiber content

1 day before	
8:00	Pursennid (Gentle Nature Ex-lax): 13 tablets, 12 mg each, taken at breakfast in one administration
13:00	lunch according to schedule
17:00	15 g of magnesium sulfate dissolved in half a glass of lukewarm water
17:30	1 glass of water or similar non carbonated beverage every 20 min up to 2 L
21:00	fast until examination
	No cleansing enemas

When it seems useful to prevent vago-vagal reflexes and to reduce colonic mucosal secretion an atropine/Buscopan association is used. Atropine sulfate, which has side-effects far greater than those of Buscopan, is administered (1.5 mg per os) 40 minutes before beginning the examination so that the maximum hypotonic and antisecretive effect is actually reached during the examination; Buscopan is administered as above. As confirmed by colon manometry investigations, with the atropine/Buscopan association, though hypotonization is not more intense than the one obtained with Buscopan alone, it lasts longer, thus allowing to complete the examination in no hurry and more easily (see Chapter 12).

Glucagon has long been abandoned because, while it is very active on colonic spasm, as demonstrated by colon manometry practically it induces no hypotonic effect on the normal colon when administered in dosages below 2 mg i.v. [3] (see Chapter 13). The administration of glucagon results in a lower distention of the rectosigmoid than Buscopan [4].

Barium suspension

Barium suspension features, required to insure a good coating of the mucosa, are analyzed in Chapter 14. The barium formulation which, in our hands, has given the best results is Polibar ACB (E-Z-EM, Westbury, NY). Barotrast (Barnes-Hind, Sunnyvale, California) has been abandoned because of the too high viscosity of the suspensions.

In Italy, Polibar ACB is supplied by the name of Prontobario Colon (Bracco, Milan) in a sterile easy-to-handle prefilled enema bag containing 400 g of micronized barium sulfate plus several additives, among which gum ghatti is very important. If the above described intestinal preparation protocol is followed, with the administration of magnesium sulfate, Polibar yields the best coating results at a 57% w/v concentration, obtained by adding 600 mL of water at body temperature to the powder preparation in the bag. Actually, the interaction between barium suspension and magnesium sulfate residues in the colon lumen seems very important (see Chapter 15). Since Mg^{++} ions are highly hydrophilic, magnesium sulfate residues take water away from the barium suspension, thus increasing viscosity and leading to a real *in vivo* "thickening", with subsequent greater density of barium particles in the mucosal coating.

The suspension is vigorously shaken manually for about 20 seconds and then allowed to rest for a few minutes. Before use, the bag is inflated. If the water is sufficiently hard, there is no foaming in the suspension. Due to suspension low viscosity (see Table 1 in Chap. 14) its introduction into the colon may take place by gravity: this is a major advantage for the lower pressure onto the colon. Pressure can be risky and poorly tolerated in patients with inflammatory colon disease. No significant amount of gas bubbles has been reported after gaseous distention of the colon lumen.

Liquid Polibar, Liquid Polibar Plus and Polibar Rapid, supplied in a ready-for-use suspension respectively with 100%, 104% and 101% w/v concentration, are not registered in Italy. When used at 1:1.5 dilution, they all perfectly integrate with the physicochemical principles of *in vivo* thickening of the Genoa technique, so that the thickness of mucosal coating and the plastic effect obtained with each of them are quite comparable to those obtained with the powder preparation.

Double contrast implementation

The patient is laid down on a lateral decubitus with his/her thighs bent against the abdomen. The enema tip is placed on the anus and, by moderate and constant pressure, driven to spontaneously penetrate into the anal canal. The use of rigid enema tips is to be avoided for their risk of damaging the posterior rectal wall.

Both Altaras (Benco, Rome) and Miller (E-Z-EM) tips [5] perfectly meet the requirements. The former (Fig. 1, left) is made of smooth plastic, with a sphere end and a second more distal sphere to stop its penetration into the ampulla recti, and with a large central hole properly gauged for easy introduction of high-density barium suspensions into the colon and for drainage. The second one (Fig. 1, right) is made of soft plastic material with ellipsoidal shaped end, large central hole and additional lateral holes.

At this point the bag with the barium suspension, placed at about 1 m above the plane where the patient is lying, is connected. The patient is now asked to turn to a prone position and the suspension is introduced under fluoroscopy control. We tend not to use enema tips with retention cuffs against incontinence. Should the patient fail to re-

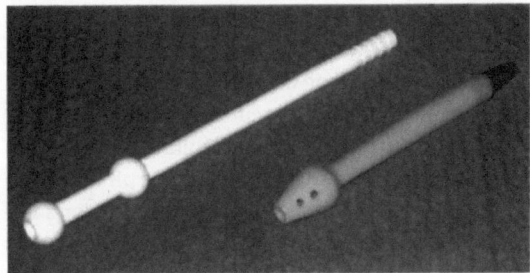

Fig. 1. Altaras' tip (Benco, Rome) (*left*) and Miller's large flexi-tip (E-Z-EM, Westbury, NY) (*right*)

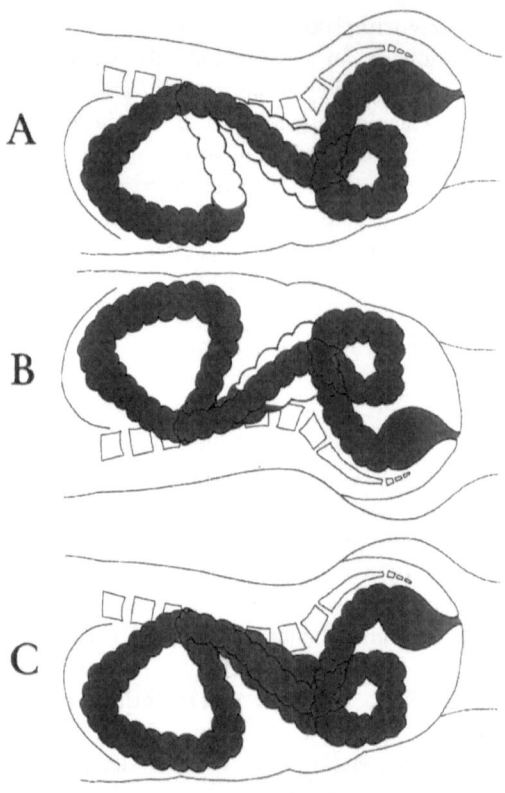

Fig. 2. Pro- and antigravity positioning of barium column, and patient's decubitus to favor barium progress. The introduction of the barium suspension starts with the patient in prone decubitus (**A**); then, as soon as the barium column slows down or stops once beyond the middle transverse colon, the patient takes a supine position (**B**), and finally takes a prone decubitus again to favor the filling of the cecum and to prevent excessive filling of the terminal ileum (**C**)

ing in a prone position (Fig. 2). Now the patient is asked to turn to the right side and lie supine: this position will favor the rapid filling of the transverse and right colon by gravity. At this point, to prevent the excessive filling of the terminal ileum, which joins the posteromedial wall of the cecum, the patient is required to rapidly take a prone position. All these postural requirements have carefully been examined by Miller [6].

The patient slowly turns around two or three times, in order to promote barium suspension contact with the colon mucosa, and then is left in a prone position. After cutting the connection between the enema tip and the bag, any surplus barium in the colon lumen is drained into a standard bowl through the rectal tip left in place. This procedure is preferred to that of draining directly into the bag, because it allows to check the drained suspension looking for any trail of mucus, blood or fecal material. The same maneuvers as in the previous filling phase are now required: starting with the patient in prone position, he/she will then be asked to slowly raise the left side and emptying will be completed in supine position. Emptying through defecation is absolutely not advisable since no exact quantification is possible.

Just before insufflation, which is done under fluoroscopy with about 2 L of air, 20 mg of Buscopan are administered i.v., as already mentioned above. The plastified rubber ball supplied as accessory by E-Z-EM is used for insufflation, by which 40 mL of air are blown with each compression. As soon as the cecum is properly distended, the enema tip is removed and a set of radiographs are taken as required by the standard procedure.

Radiographic technique

The examination is normally performed on a tipping table with TV remote fluoroscopic control. For the radiographic technique, high voltage (120 kVp), short exposure time (0.02-0.04 s), fine focal spot (0.6 x 0.6 mm), 120-cm SID, 12:1 ratio Bucky grid, and 600-speed screen/film combinations are required.

A rigorously *standardized sequence* of 7 basic radiographs is taken to document the opposite walls of the various colon segments in dependent and nondependent position, alternatively (Table 2 and Figs. 3,4). As to the sequence, the Genoa technique

tain the barium suspension, we simply lower the bag onto the floor, wait for a few minutes and then try again bringing the bag back to the starting position.

The ampulla recti is generally filled up almost instantaneously by the barium column which, once overcome the resistance of Moutier's sphincter (see Chapter 5), flushes the sigmoid and easily flows upward along the descending colon. It then slows down progressively and sometimes stops once beyond the left flexure because of the antigravity position of the transverse colon when the patient is ly-

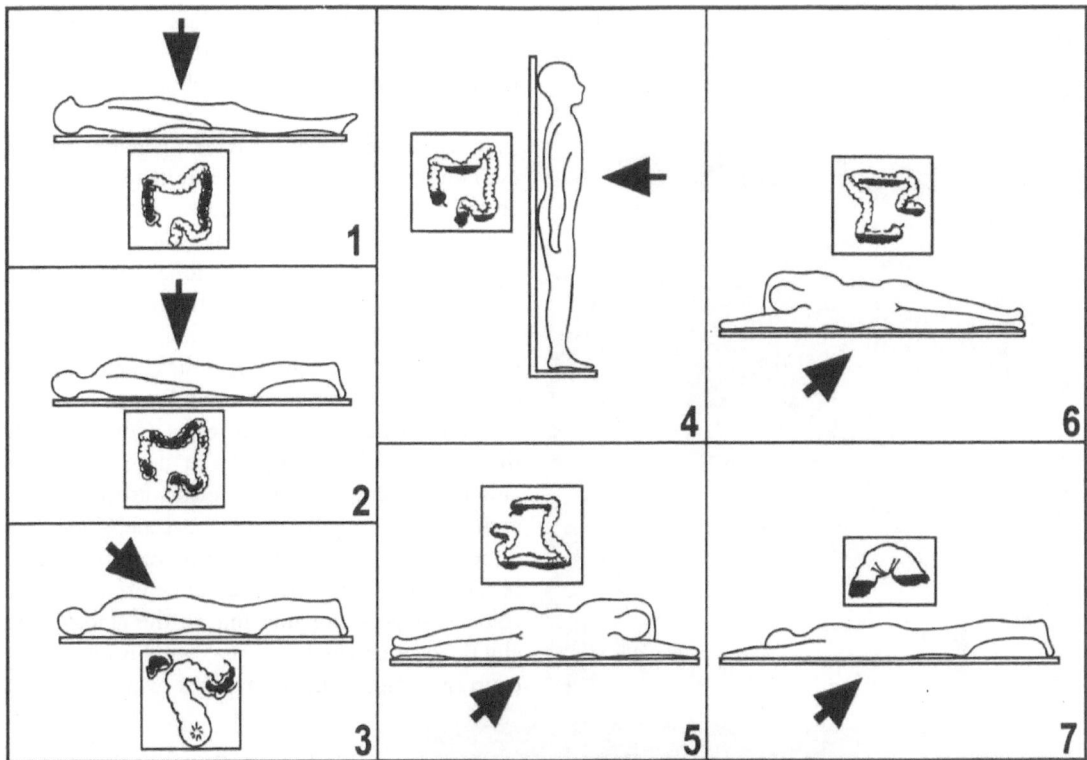

Fig. 3. The 3 stages in the standard radiographic sequence proposed by the Genoa technique. **1**, **2** and **3**: horizontally positioned radiographic table; **4**: vertically positioned radiographic table; **5**, **6** and **7**: radiographs taken with the patient lying on an accessory table close to the vertically positioned radiographic table. See also Table 2 and Fig. 4

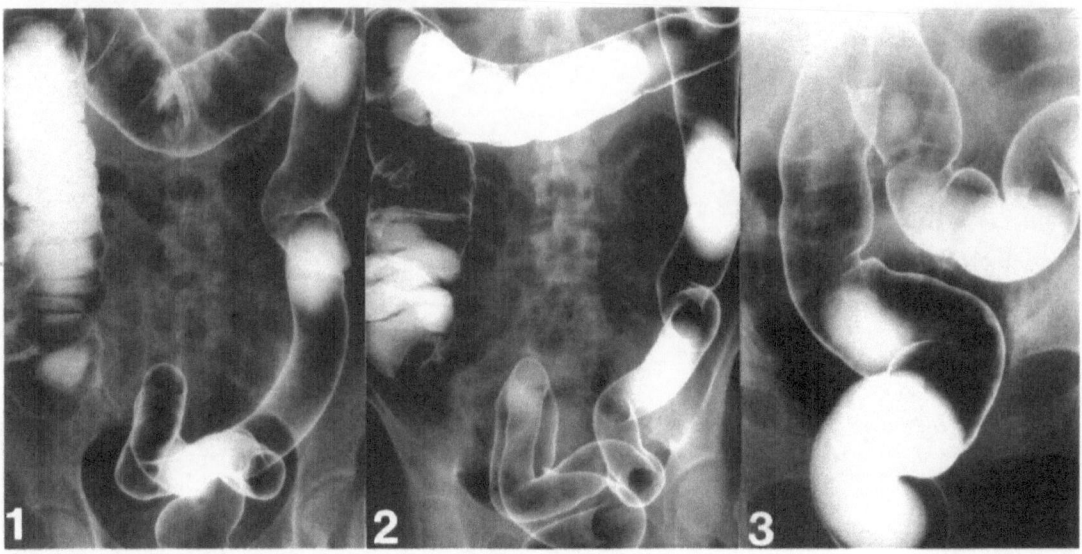

Fig. 4. The 7 basic radiographs of the Genoa technique. See also Fig. 3

(cont.)

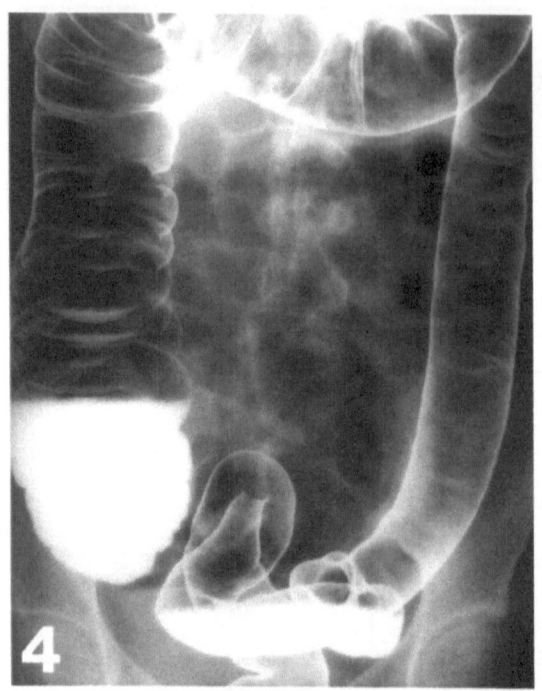

is significantly different from the radiographic sequence proposed by Welin and Welin [7] (Fig. 5), as well as that by Altaras [8] defined as "colon status" (Fig. 6).

A brief examination of the radiographs will tell the radiologist whether the examination – lasting, on the whole, about 20 minutes – can be considered completed, or additional spot radiographs or different views may be required for a thorough documentation of any pathological finding.

In double-contrast examination, image contrast is intrinsically very high due to the concurrent presence of a great amount of air and mucosal coating with high density barium particles. Contrast is further increased by the significant difference in size among the various colon segments as well as their arrangement along different planes and slopes with respect to the X-ray beam. This poses a considerable obstacle to the concurrent accurate exposure of all colon segments and therefore to the global "readability" of each single image. For this reason, low contrast radiography is required which, as men-

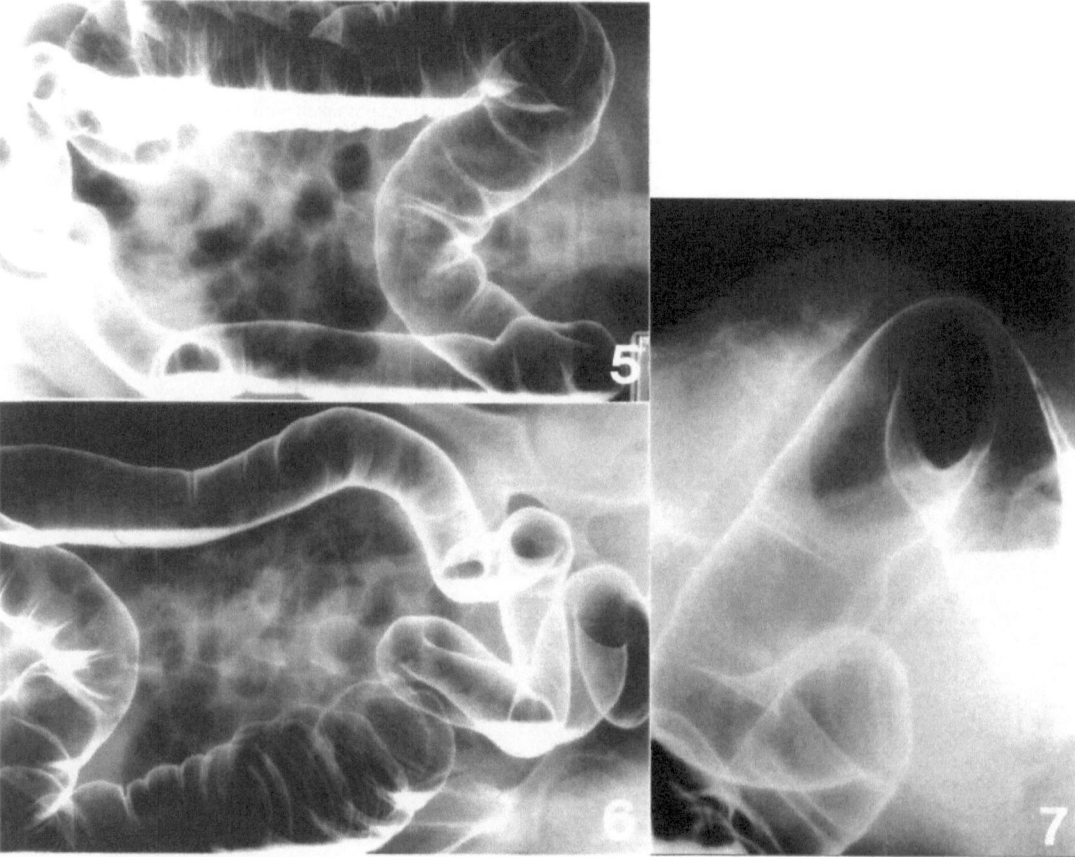

Fig. 4. (continued)

Table 2. DCBE: the radiographic sequence

X-ray tube	Cassette	Projection	Patient
1. Vertical	14" x 17"	AP	supine
2. Vertical	14" x 17"	PA	prone
3. Angled 40° caudally	14" x 17"	PA	prone
4. Horizontal	14" x 17"	AP	upright
5. Horizontal	14" x 17"	AP	left lateral decubitus on a table close to the vertically positioned radiographic table
6. Horizontal	14" x 17"	AP	as in 5 but with the patient in right lateral decubitus
7. Horizontal	10" x 12"	LL	as in 5 but with the patient prone (field of view limited to the rectosigmoid)

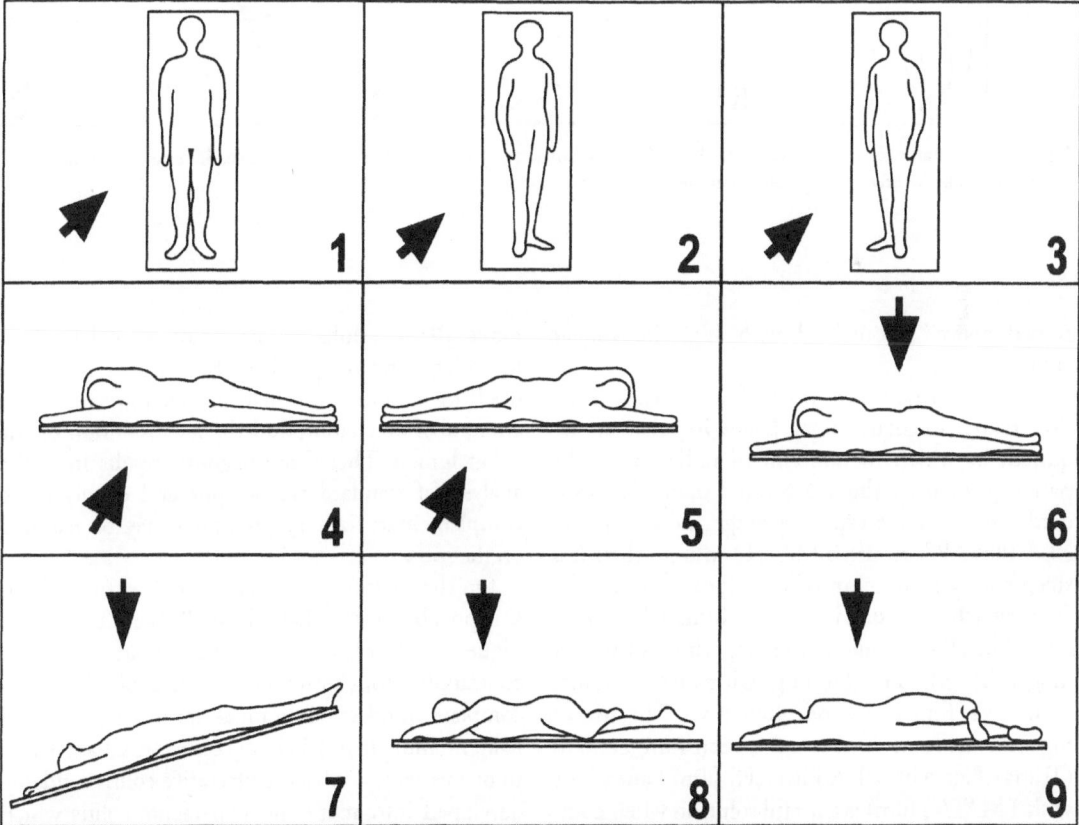

Fig. 5. The standard radiographic sequence proposed by Welin and Welin [7]. **1, 2** and **3**: vertically positioned radiographic table; **4** and **5**: radiographs taken on the accessory table; **6, 7, 8** and **9**: radiographs taken on the horizontally positioned radiographic table

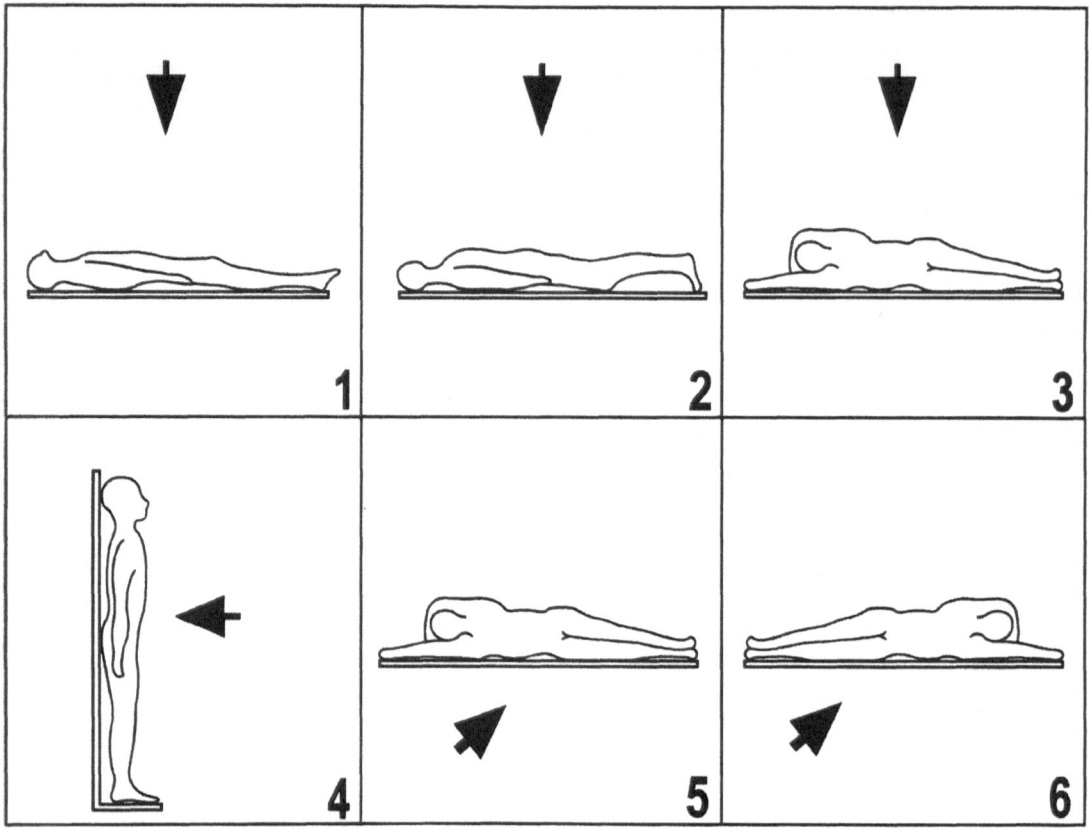

Fig. 6. "Colon status" according to Altaras [8]. **1**, **2** and **3**: horizontally positioned radiographic table; **4**: vertically positioned radiographic table; **5** and **6**: radiographs taken on the accessory table

tioned above, is obtained with high kilovoltage equipment.

High speed rare earth intensifying screens (Imation Trimax Regular; Kodak Lanex Regular) are required, by which the amount of radiation to the patient is reduced about 4-6 times than with standard screens. Wide exposure range films (Imation XLA Plus APS; Kodak TMAT/L), due to their less steep contrast slope can offset minor exposure defects, which with standard range films (XDA Plus APS; TMAT/G) would require repetition of the radiographs [9]. The Sterling UltraVision system with UVL film is a good alternative. The use of higher resolution low speed screen/film systems (Trimax Fine with XDA Plus APS film; Lanex Fine with TMAT/G film) is a useful solution when complementary detail radiographs are needed.

For X-ray protection reasons (see Chapter 17) the use of fluoroscopy is very limited in the Genoa technique. Besides, unlike SCBE, fluoroscopy has a limited diagnostic role in DCBE, where it is mainly used to monitor the barium column flow, the amount of evacuation and the air distention of the colon lumen. Therefore, diagnosis results from the analysis of standard radiographs and of any other complementary radiograph which may be required on the spot.

On the basis of more than 41,000 examinations, it is possible to say that, all in all, the Genoa technique is well tolerated. Pediatric or old age are no contraindications to its use. About 25% of patients complain modest abdominal localized or spread pain; no more than 7% have colics (see Chapter 10). In one patient, a subacute ulcerative colitis suddenly developed into acute and hyperacute colitis which required immediate surgery. Two patients at the beginning of the examination had a subperitoneal perforation of the posterior wall of the rectum.

It must be stressed that in the Genoa technique each choice, no matter if shared or not, has its own motivation and it has often resulted from the failure or shortcomings of the other previous choices. Every personal change which seems logical to introduce, when practically tested, often clashes against unexpected obstacles. This is a further confirmation, if it were necessary, that DCBE is an extremely delicate technique to implement.

References

1. Cittadini G, Rollandi GA, Russo S (1986) Intestino crasso. In: Cittadini G, Tecnica di studio a doppio contrasto del tubo digerente: la via italiana. Genova: Ecig, pp. 89-110
2. Cittadini G, Rollandi GA, Giribaldi M (1980) Su un metodo semplice innocuo ed efficiente di pulizia intestinale senza clisteri. Radiol Med 66:415-420
3. Oliva L, Cittadini G (1981) Il clisma a doppio contrasto: problemi metodologici e tecnici. Verona: Cortina, pp. 106.
4. Goei R, Nix M, Kessels AH, Ten Tusscher MP (1995) Use of antispasmodic drugs in double contrast barium enema examination: glucagon or buscopan? Clin Radiol 50:553-557
5. Miller RE (1969) A new enema tip. Radiology 92:1492
6. Miller RE (1979) Solution for the "Air block" problem during fluoroscopy. AJR 132:1020-1021
7. Welin S, Welin G (1976) The double contrast examination of the colon. Experience with the Welin modification. Stuttgart: Thieme
8. Altaras J (1982) Radiologischer Atlas, Kolon und Rektum. München: Urban & Schwarzenberg
9. Rollandi GA, Gambaro A, Pulzato P et al (1984) Utilizzazione di una pellicola a basso gradiente di contrasto nelle indagini a doppio contrasto del tubo digerente. Radiol Med 70(Suppl 4):89-91

5   Fundamentals of large bowel anatomy related to the problems of DCBE

In this chapter, several aspects of the large bowel macro- and microscopic anatomy will be considered which acquire particular importance when carrying out the DCBE procedure and for its interpretation, namely:

- the three-dimensional lay-out of the various colon segments, which affects barium and air collection depending on patient's decubitus;
- the ileocecal valve, which may either take a dependent or nondependent position with respect to its attachment in the cecum, thus affecting proper barium filling of the last ileal loop;
- the morphology of the semilunar folds and the haustral pouches [1], which becomes important in the assessment of impaired colon motility;
- the colon sphincters;
- the innominate grooves.

The sympathetic and parasympathetic innervation of the large intestine will be described in Chapter 11.

The large bowel varies from 150 to 180 cm in length, about one fourth of the small intestine. Its caliber narrows progressively from 6 cm in the cecum and transverse colon, to 2-3 cm in the distal portion of the sigmoid and increases again in the rectum. Its shape varies depending on constitutional habit and age: it is round, O-shaped in brachymorphic individuals and children, whereas it is vaguely M-shaped in the elderly and longilineal individuals. It features six segments: the cecum, the ascending colon, the transverse colon, the descending colon, the sigmoid colon and the rectum (Fig. 1).

The **cecum** takes an oblique position from the front to the back and from the bottom to the top (fig. 5.1). It is 6-8 cm high with a cross-sectional diameter of approximately 6 cm. The appendix branches off from the lower portion of the cecum, where also the taeniae coli originate. Conventionally, a horizontal plane passing across the highest portion of the ileocecal sphincter is considered to be the upper limit of the cecum. Normally, it is totally enfolded by the peritoneum; therefore, it can be moved quite easily. However, the degree of mobility depends on the posterior peritoneal attachment of the cecum. Morphological variations are common depending on the level of posterior peritoneal reflection.

The **ascending colon** has a slightly smaller caliber than the cecum. It runs obliquely upwards and backwards becoming deeper as it approaches the right flexure. It averages about 8 to 12 cm in length. The peritoneal serosa, which runs from the lateral wall of the abdominal cavity to the posterior wall, covers the ascending colon anteriorly, while its posterior side lies above the quadratus lumborum muscle facing the retroperitoneal space. It can thus be considered as a fixed segment.

The **right flexure** is located between the ascending and the transverse colon, forming an angle which opens caudally, anteriorly and to the interior. It lies quite deep inside.

Since the right hepatic flexure is more caudal than the left colic flexure, the **transverse colon** ascends across the abdominal cavity, along a ventrally convex arch. Its central part lies more anteriorly than the two sides. It is approximately 50

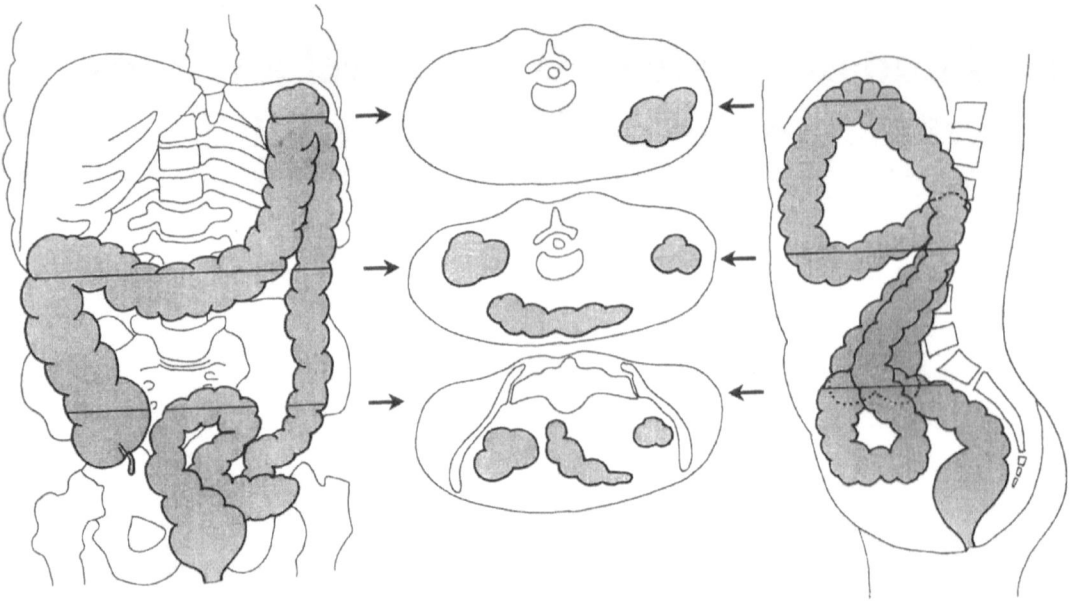

Fig. 1. Three-dimensional layout of the various colon segments. *Left*: frontal view; *Center*: the three fundamental cross-section levels (from top to bottom, the splenic flexure, the lower segment of the transverse colon, the angle between descending and ascending segments of the sigmoid); *Right*: left lateral view, displaying the double ring image induced by the transverse and sigmoid colon

cm long. It is attached to the posterior abdominal wall by a peritoneal fold, the transverse mesocolon, which gives the colon a considerable range of movement: when going from supine decubitus to standing position, the transverse colon may sag down some distance from its central abdominal position down to the pubic symphysis.

The **left flexure**, situated between the transverse and the descending colon, forms an acute angle, the medial side of which, the ascending one, is more anterior, and the lateral descending one runs posteriorly, yet at a lower depth than the descending colon. Since the left flexure is more anterior than the right one, when the patient is prone, the barium suspension, having easily run through the rectum, the sigmoid, the descending and the splenic flexure, stops here due to the antigravity position of the transverse colon. By changing the patient from prone to supine position, the barium enema will then be able to flow across the transverse and the right flexure (see Fig. 2 in Chap. 4).

The **descending colon**, some 12 to 20 cm in length, extends downward from the left colic flex-

ure to the iliac crest. It runs more or less vertically and quite posteriorly. Like the ascending colon, only its anterior surface is covered by the peritoneum, while its posterior surface faces the retroperitoneal space on the quadratus lumborum muscle. It is therefore a fixed segment.

The **sigmoid**, conventionally limited by the descending colon along a horizontal plane across the iliac crest, runs downward and sometimes even rightward. Depending on its position with the peritoneum, it can be distinguished into an upper iliac portion, without mesentery and thus fixed, which follows a slightly downward, inward and backward concave curve, and a lower pelvic portion with a more or less long mesentery allowing it to move freely inside the pelvis minor. This portion assumes an inverted U-shaped flexure arching over the pelvic inlet to finally join the rectum at the level of the third sacral vertebra. However, due to different arrangements of the mesosigmoid, the length and shape of the sigmoid may vary considerably. According to Farrar [2], despite wide variations, the sigmoid can be radiologically distinguished into five segments

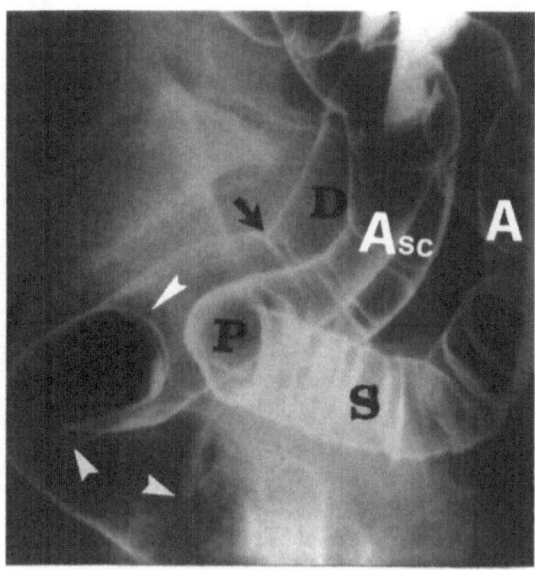

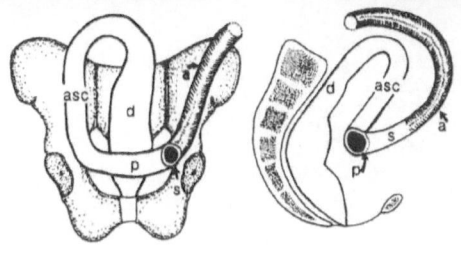

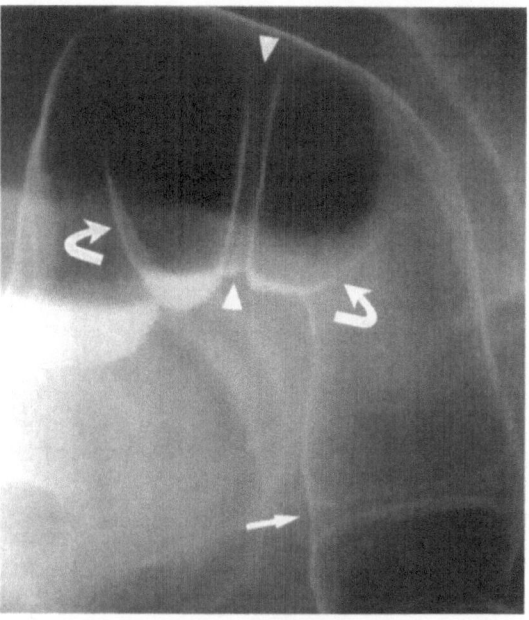

Fig. 3. In a rectum detail in lateral projection, the Kohlrausch fold (*arrowhead*), which is perpendicularly hit by the X-ray beam, takes up a peculiar "railway track" appearance (see Fig. 10). The upper and lower Houston folds (*curved arrows*), obliquely hit by the X-ray beam, resemble bow-like lines. The Strauss fold (*straight arrows*) should be noted, marking the passage from the rectum to the descending segment of the sigmoid

Fig. 2. The five segments of the sigmoid according to Farrar [2]. From bottom to top: D = descending; ASC = ascending; P = posterior; S = superior; A = anterior. *Arrowheads* = lower Houston fold, Kohlrausch fold, upper Houston fold. *Black arrow* = Strauss fold. See also Fig. 3.

(Fig. 2) which, from bottom to top, are the following: descending sigmoid, which joins the rectum; ascending, parallel to the former one and located anteriorly; posterior, with a right to left transversal arrangement; superior, obliquely running to the front and upward; anterior, running vertically toward the descending colon.

The **rectum** extends from the third sacral vertebra down to the anorectal line. Depending on its position with respect to the pelvic peritoneum, it can be distinguished into a superior, retroperitoneal pelvic portion and an inferior, subperitoneal perineal portion. Actually the peritoneum, after covering the bladder (and, in the female, the body of the uterus), moves forward to the anterior wall of the rectum where it reflects upward covering only the upper portion. The pelvic portion, about 12-14 cm long, conforms to the sacral curve from which it is separated by the rectosacral space. The perineal portion, which is situated more anterior but with a sharp backward turn, is 7-8 cm in length.

Some interesting rectal structures can be shown directly with DCBE (Fig. 3), namely: the *Houston folds*, mucosal folds located to the right and left side of the ampulla recti; the *Kohlrausch fold*, a median semilunar mucosal relief which is found – but not always – in between the previous folds; the *semilunar terminal Strauss fold*, at the border of the rectosigmoid junction; the *columns and sinuses of Morgagni* which, in variable number from 5 to 10, are arranged along the circumference of the rectum on its more distal portion (Fig. 4).

The ileocecal valve is located in the posteromedial wall of the cecum. (Fig. 5). For this reason the patient should be placed in a prone position as soon as the barium suspension reaches

31

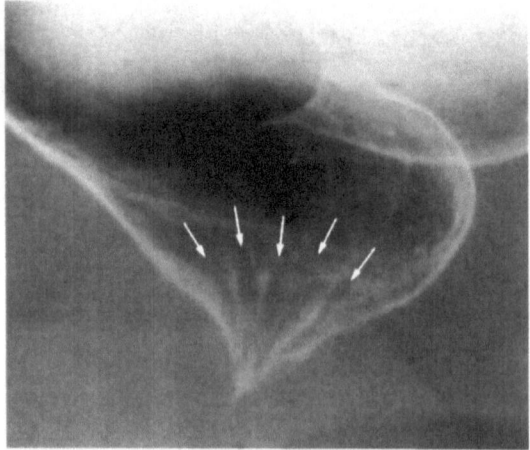

Fig. 4. Morgagni's columns and sinuses, which are penetrated by the barium suspension, form a sunburst pattern converging on the anal canal (*arrows*)

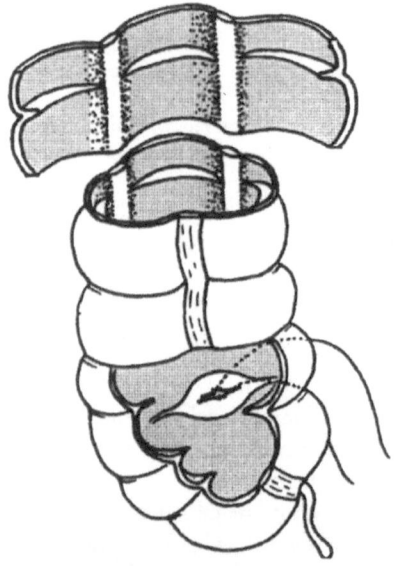

Fig. 5. Internal and external outline of the right colon. The inlet of the last ileal fold should be noted, which is more or less medial to the posterior wall of the cecum

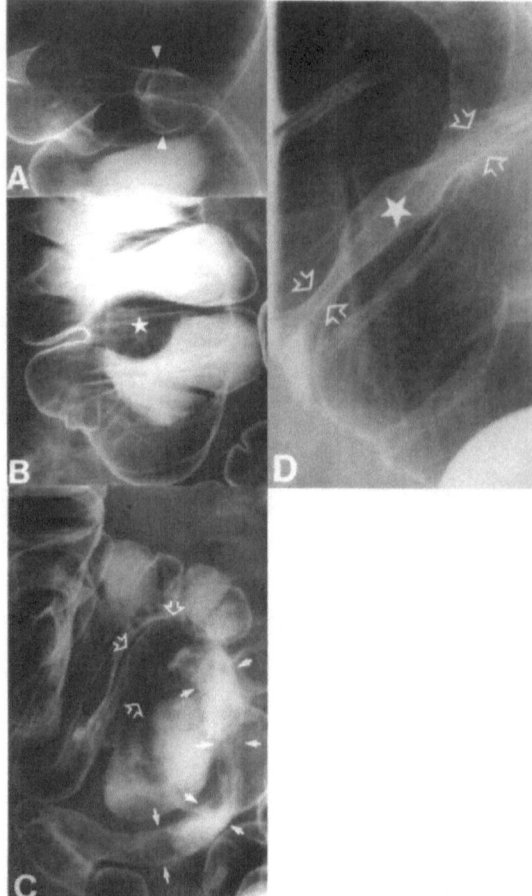

Fig. 6. Three different aspects of the ileocecal valve. (**A**), round-shaped endocecal tumefaction directly visible on the double-contrast image (*arrowheads*); (**B**), round-shaped endocecal filling defect visible on the barium pool when the patient lies supine (*star*); (**C**), like (B) (*open arrows*), but with barium-filled star-like central opening (*arrows*); (**D**) transversally oblong tumefaction (*star*) stretching between the two frenula (*arrows*)

the cecum in order to prevent it from flowing into the last ileal loop. In the living individual, the ileocecal valve has a papillary form, with a small round or starlike central opening, or is transversally slightly elongated. With the DCBE, this papillary shape is directly demonstrated when the X-ray beam is uprightly driven through it, looking like a roundish endocecal tumefaction (Fig. 6A-C). Similar findings are also recorded in case of a more or less pronounced invagination of the

terminal ileum into the cecum. More commonly, however, due to the type of projection, it looks like a transversally oblong tumefaction with perfectly clear-cut and regular margins (Fig. 6D).

With DCBE the colonic folds and the haustral pouches can be demonstrated directly. Since this demonstration has recently become important for the X-ray assessment of some colonic motility alterations (see Chapter 19), it is necessary to examine the anatomic substrate which was particularly investigated by Meyers [3, 4] (Fig. 5).

The three taeniae (the taenia omentalis, libera

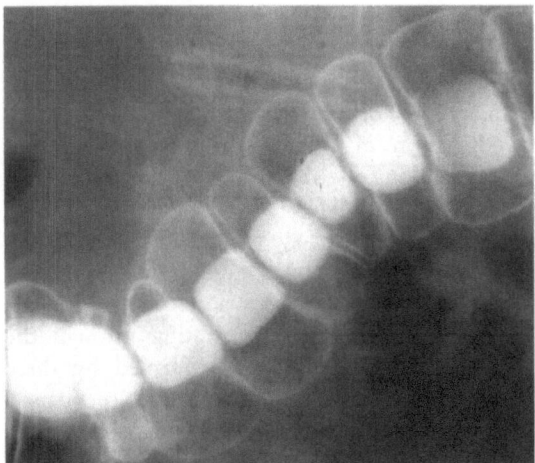

Fig. 7. Clover-like sacculations (see text). When the patient is supine, the posterior sacculation of the transverse colon is well demonstrated by the barium collection

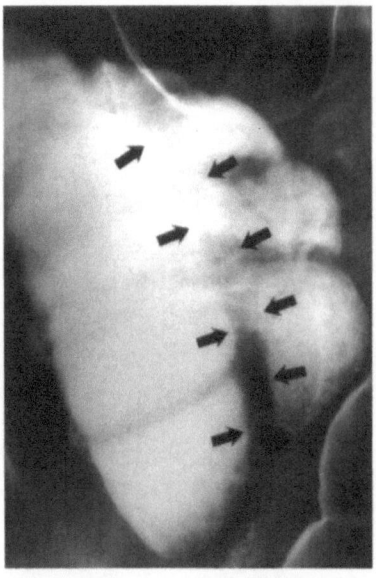

Fig. 9. Ribbon-like filling defect (*arrows*) induced by the anterior taenia in the ascending colon and in the cecum which are partially distended by the barium suspension

and mesocolica), where the longitudinal muscles thicken into bands, run along the total length of the colon. These, being shorter than the colon and with greater contractile tone, help to shape the external colon surface into bulges, which are more numerous in the right and transverse colon, and separated by angular furrows arranged transversally to the major colon axis.

The internal colonic lumen is the negative image of the external surface. The external bulges correspond to the haustra, while the angular furrows correspond to the plicae semilunares, which are proper anatomic formations constituted by mucosa, submucosa and muscle layer. They protrude into the colonic lumen by about 6-8 mm.

The arrangement of the taeniae – one of which is always anterior (the taenia omentalis in the cecum and the ascending colon, and the free taenia in the transverse colon), while the other two are posterior (medio-lateral in the cecum-ascending and the descending colon; cranio-caudal in the transverse colon) – subdivides each haustral pouch into "clover-like" sacculations. When the patient is supine, small pools of barium collect in the posterior sacculation, thus forming X-ray images like the one in Fig. 7.

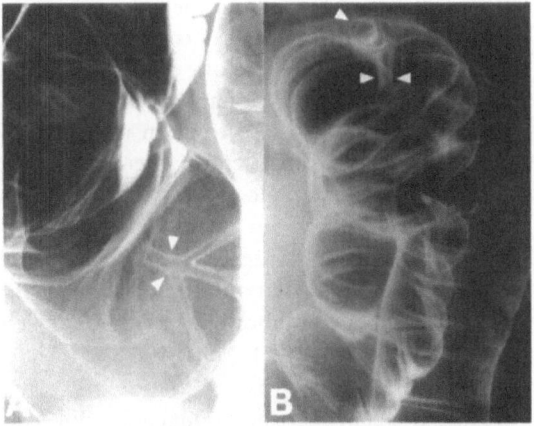

Fig. 8. Two uncommon features of the taeniae (*arrowheads*), seen by transparency in the double-contrast images of the fundus of the cecum (**A**) and of the left flexure(**B**)

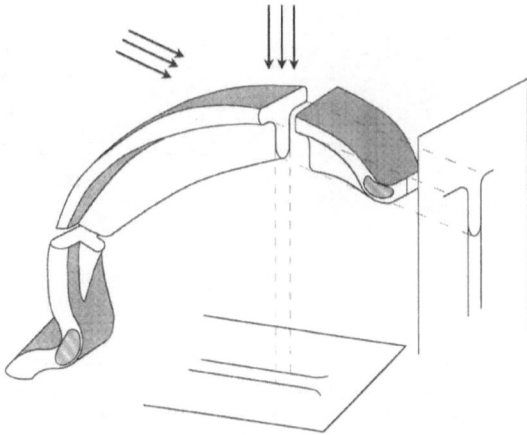

Fig. 10. "Rail-track" and "hair-pin" appearance of the semilunar fold (see text)

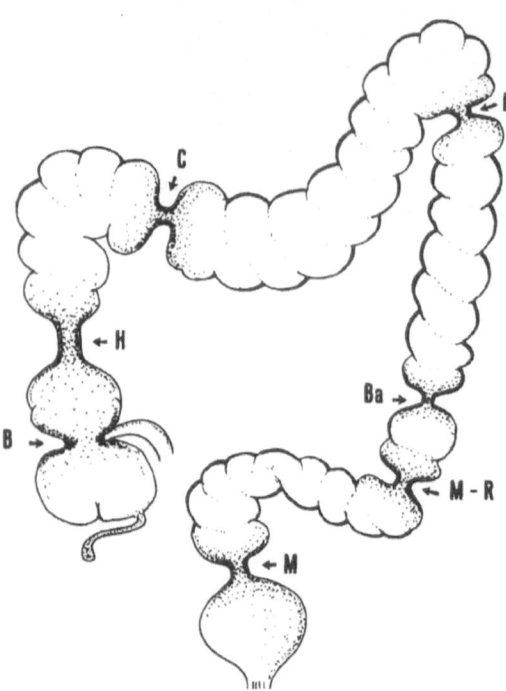

Fig. 11. Pseudo-sphincters of the colon. From the rectum towards the cecum: Moutier, Moutier-Rossi, Balli, Payr, Cannon, Hirsch and Busi sphincter

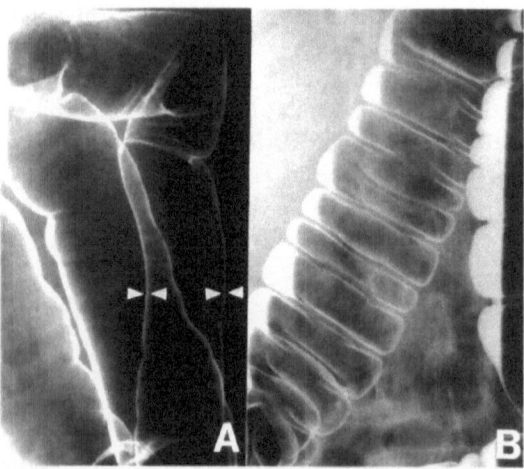

Fig. 12. (A), the mucosal surface, which is tangentially hit by the X-ray beam, appears like a more or less intensely radiopaque line (*arrowheads*); in the space between these marginal lines, a uniform medium-gray veil is formed by the overlapping projection of dependent and nondependent mucosal surfaces. (B), semilunar folds, identifiable by their peculiar "railtrack" appearance, are arranged transversally to the major colon axis: more or less long, they divide the colon lumen into several haustral pouches

The taeniae can be said to originate in the furrow along the cecum contour where the appendix joins the cecum. The direct demonstration of taeniae, for short portions, is much less common, in the form of thin, slightly opaque ribbons arranged along the major axis of the colon (Fig. 8) or of filling defects (Fig. 9), if observed by DC or SC, respectively.

The semicircular folds extend along one portion of the circumference of each loop. The barium suspension, when penetrating through the two opposite dihedral angles formed by these folds together with the mucosal surface, depicts a thin radiopaque line on both sides of their image. In this way, the normal fold, when seen upright, looks like a rail, when seen from the profile it looks like a hair-pin inprinting the edge of the colon (Fig. 10). The semilunar folds which are numerous in the right colon, progressively diminish in numbers toward the sigmoid.

Controversial speculations about the presence of pseudo-sphincters (Fig. 11) scattered along the colon were advanced in the past. In his ad-hoc investigations, Balli [5] was able to observe that only in the case of the sphincters of Busi, Hirsch and Moutier can muscle-nerve relations be observed as different from the other parts of the colon. With personal manometric investigations up to 60 cm from the anal verge, we have observed a hyperpressure area of 2-3 cm in length at the level of the rectosigmoid junction in the alleged site of Moutier's sphincter where, actually, a temporary stop of the barium column is generally observed on X-ray examination.

With the barium coating, the colonic mucosa looks as covered by a homogeneous medium-gray carpet when seen "en face" by the X-ray beam, whereas it takes the appearance of an intensely radiopaque line when seen from an upright view (Fig. 12). This standard picture, where dependent and nondependent mucosal surfaces are seen through each other, can be obtained for each colonic segment in those standard spots where the colon is in antigravity position as against the adjacent segments. Otherwise, a more or less large barium pool will be observed on the dependent surface (Fig. 13).

The surface of the colonic mucosa, unlike the stomach, is smooth. This facilitates the detection of pathologic conditions even of few millimeters in size. However, sometimes, in SC or DC spots,

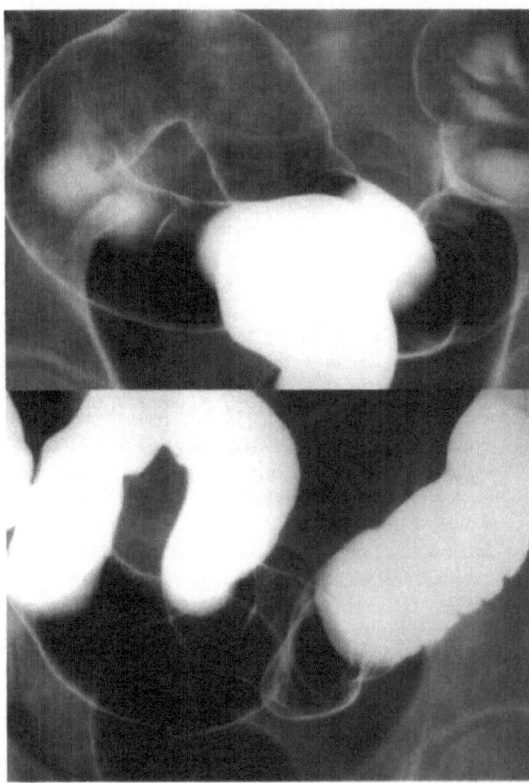

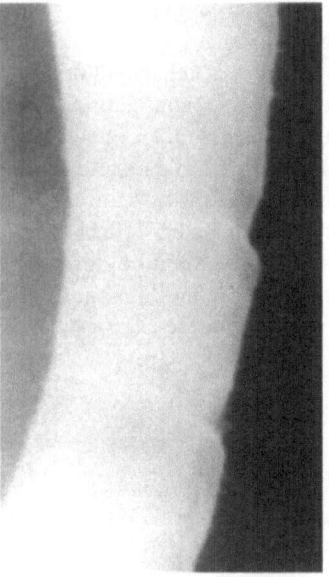

Fig. 14. The innominate grooves. In the single-contrast image they often look like fine protrusions of the colon profile looking like tapered spicules

Fig. 13. Detail of the sigmoid colon. It should be noted that in going from supine (*top*) to prone decubitus (*bottom*), the double-contrast image of nondependent surfaces becomes a barium collection image, and viceversa for dependent surfaces

kVp recommended voltage). The innominate lines can be demonstrated in 89% of cases (in 33% for the whole colon and 56% in individual portions).

it is possible to observe fine protrusions of the colon profile looking like tapered spicules, at 1-3 mm intervals from each other and 0.5-1 mm deep (Fig. 14). Today, this finding is considered to be the expression of the innominate lines [6,7], but in the past it was mistaken for colitic erosions or intramural diverticuli, or later wrongly attributed to the barium filling of the Lieberkuhn's glands [8]. In DC images, the innominate lines seen "en face" give the mucosal surface a finely dotted or meshed appearance (Fig. 15) (See also Fig. 10 in Chap. 3).

A good demonstration of the innominate lines depends on DCBE implementation technique [9]. Particularly important are intestinal preparation (a proper diet and laxatives without cleansing enemas is the best approach) and the characteristics of the barium suspension (with concentration of approximately 65% w/v for best results), as well as the radiographic technique (100

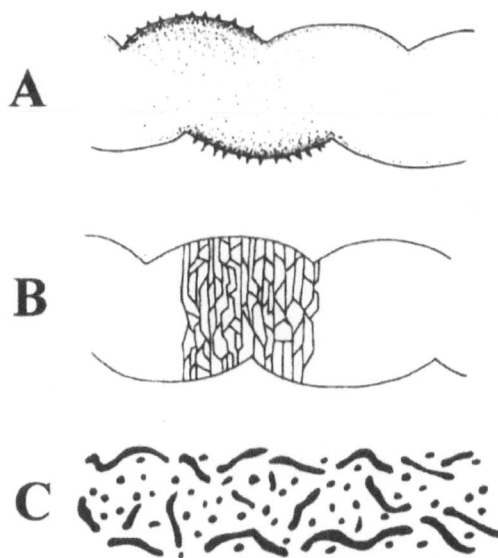

Fig. 15. Schematic drawing of the most common radiological appearances of the innominate grooves according to Williams [6] (**A**), marginal tapered spicules; (**B**), reticular; (**C**), linear and punctate

The presence of the innominate lines, which is a constant finding in anatomic specimens, is connected to the presence, at regular intervals, of lymphoid aggregates which account for the contracture of the muscularis mucosae: the overlying mucosa, thinner and without glands and mucine producing cells, is stretched, thus forming regularly scattered surface depressions [10,11].

Studies of the behavior of the innominate lines during early ulcerative and granulomatous colitis have so far failed to yield interesting results.

References

1. Weissman A, Bousquet J-C, Harriague D et al (1980) Aspects de l'anatomie radiologique du côlon en double contraste. J Radiol Electrol Med Nucl 61:301-311
2. Farrar CW (1979) Patterns of sigmoid colon and their implications for barium-enema radiography. Med Radiogr Photogr 55/1:2-28
3. Meyers MA, Volberg F, Katzen B et al (1973) Haustral anatomy and pathology: A new look. I. Roentgen identification of normal pattern and relationships. Radiology 108:497-504
4. Meyers MA, Volberg F, Katzen B et al. Haustral anatomy and pathology: A new look. II. Roentgen interpretation of pathological alterations. Radiology 1973; 108:505-512
5. Balli R (1948) Semeiotica e diagnostica röntgen. Milano: Wassermann & C. Vol II, pp 67-75
6. Williams I (1965) Innominate grooves in the surface of the mucosa. Radiology 84:877-880
7. Frank DF, Berk RN, Goldstein HM (1977) Pseudoulcerations of the colon on barium enema examination. Gastrointest Radiol 2:129-131
8. Dassel PM (1962) Innocuous filling of the intestinal glands of the colon durinmg barium enema (spiculation) simulating organic disease. Radiology 78:799-801
9. Cole FM (1978) Innominate grooves of the colon: morphological characteristics and etiologic mechanisms. Radiology 128:41-42
10. Matsuura K, Nakata H, Takeda N et al (1977) Innominate lines of the colon. Radiology 123:581-584
11. Ruffato C, Liessi G, Valente R et al (1979) Kritische betrachtungen zu den "innominate grooves" des kolons. Fortschr Geb Rontgenstr Nuklearmed 131:594-599

6 Fundamentals of large bowel physiology related to the problems of DCBE

In a modern radiological approach to the study of large bowel diseases starting from the technical implementation of individual examinations, a deep knowledge of the physiology and physiopathology of the intestine is required. For example, the DCBE technique involves a preparatory phase followed by the implementation of the proper examination, during which maneuvers are carried out that may alter the physiologic balance of the large bowel. Cleansing enemas, laxatives of various types, the injection into the colon of barium mixed with air, lead all to major motor and metabolic changes which the radiologist cannot neglect. Therefore, before examining each of them in detail, we shall first examine some basic physiopathologic concepts of the large bowel, with the aim to better evaluate the mutual impact between radiological examination and the most important functions of the colon: absorption, excretion, secretion, intestinal flora activity and motility (Table 1).

Absorption and excretion

Discussing colon absorption without mentioning excretion, would only be a partial approach to the issue. Indeed, the amount of absorbed and excreted substances (H_2O, Na^+, Cl^-, K^+, HCO_3^-, NH_4^+, volatile fatty acids, glucides, protides) results out of a constant flow from and to the lumen regulated by active and passive transport mechanisms at constant osmolarity.

Table 1. Colon functions

1. *Absorption*
   H_2O Na^+ Cl^- carbohydrates lipids proteins

2. *Excretion*
   K^+ HCO_3^- NH_4^+

3. *Secretion*
   seric proteins (alpha and beta globulins), enzymes (lysozyme, etc.), mucus

4. *Intestinal flora activities*

5. *Motor activities*

The colon absorbs sodium, chloride, and mainly water (Table 2). 120-125 mEq/L daily of sodium reach the colon, while approximately 25-50 mEq/L leave the intestine with the feces: hence, a healthy individual with a daily evacuation containing 100 mL of water eliminates about 3 mEq of sodium.

Table 2. H_2O, Na^+ and Cl^- absorption

- The daily amount of H_2O absorbed by the colon is 900-1,400 mL

- Colon potential water absorption amounts to 5-7 L/day, i.e. 5-6 times greater than actual physiologic absorption

- Sodium absorption capacity of the colon is 4-5 times greater than any other segment of the digestive tract

Sodium was calculated to be absorbed by the colonic mucosa at a rate of 0.28 mEq/min [1]. This means that, when a continuous isotonic saline perfusion is administered, the colon is capable of reabsorbing up to 400 mEq/day of sodium, corresponding to one sixth of extracellular sodium. Therefore, the large bowel potential absorption is 7 times greater than its actual physiologic absorption, and is fully exploited when the colon undergoes powerful stimuli, such as repeated enemas or hypertonic infusions [2].

Sodium is absorbed through active transport linked with the sodium pump and regulated by the Na/K dependent adenosine-triphosphatase, against a steep concentration gradient (starting from a mere 15 mEq/L concentration in the lumen and with a 40 mV potential difference with a negative intestinal wall) [3]. Sodium is passively transported from the lumen to the wall when its concentration in the lumen exceeds 75 mEq/L.

The colon absorbs 0.39 mEq/L of chlorides. Electrochemical gradients alone are responsible for the transfer of chlorides from the lumen to the intestinal wall, then flowing into the blood only through a passive transport mechanism.

Potassium and bicarbonates are the main substances excreted by the colon (Table 3). In the colonic mucosa, the potassium flow direction is opposite to that of the sodium. Potassium has a one-direction flow to the intestinal lumen at a 0.03 mEq/min speed. In case of continuous perfusion, up to 32 mEq/day of potassium can be lost.

Table 3. K^+ and HCO_3^- excretion

• A biologic Na/K pump is working in the colon for active sodium transport from the lumen to the wall, and for potassium transport in the opposite direction

• Under constant perfusion, the potential loss of potassium is extremely high in the colon

• Repeated colon washing with enemas or peroral wash-outs are comparable with continuous perfusion

---

The potassium flow from the wall to the colonic lumen is either passive, following electrochemical gradients [4], or takes place through the Na/K pump [5]. The concurrent active transport of sodium from the lumen to the wall and that of potassium in the opposite direction, in order to maintain an electrolytic balance, is ensured by the Na/K pump.

HCO_3^- also flows from the intestinal wall to the lumen. Under certain conditions (for example, acidosis) this flow can take the opposite direction. However, it is always passively transported at a rate of 0.18 mEq/min.

Water uptake needs to be discussed in greater detail. Every day the colon receives 1,000-1,500 mL of isotonic pH 6-7 chyme from the ileum and it expels about 150 g of feces (30 g of solids and 120 g of water). Therefore, the colon absorbs about 900-1,400 mL/day of water, 85-90% of which in the right colon [6]. These data are in contrast with those maintaining that the colon is the water-saving organ of the digestive system. The 900-1,400 mL of water absorbed by the large bowel is very little compared to the 8,000 mL absorbed by the small intestine, not to mention its water saving potential.

Yet, water transport, absorption and excretion physiology is not so simple. The large intestine is indeed well known to be the organ with the highest blood flow (0.92 mL/g/min) in the human body, with a daily flow of 1,000 liters of blood [7]. With this property, the water exchanged between the blood compartment and the intestinal lumen exceeds 18 L/day; therefore, the 900-1,400 mL of apparently absorbed water do not simply derive from mucus absorption, but originate from complex hydroelectric mechanisms taking place between the blood compartment and the intestinal lumen.

Based on the above mentioned blood flow rates, and assuming that, under normal conditions, the colon absorbs 900-1,400 mL/day of water, it can be inferred that its maximum capacity is 5-7 L/day [8], namely about 5-6 times greater than its actual physiologic absorption.

The hydroelectric exchange (and therefore absorption and excretion) between the contents of the colonic lumen and the blood compartment depends on functional needs of the whole body. When, due to repeated cleansing enemas, this balance is upset, the onset of pathologic conditions is likely to take place. It is extremely interesting to note that these alterations, paradoxically enough, are caused by one of the most important physiologic properties of the colon, namely its remarkable absorption and excretion capacity. For example, a constantly perfused colon can lose up to 32 mEq/day of potassium. A person hit by cholera, can lose up to 10-12 L of water daily, which means a loss of 1,500-1,600 mEq of sodium and 230-250 mEq of potassium.

From the above concepts, which are briefly summarized in Tables 2 and 3, some considerations can be made which are particularly important for the radiologist. Repeated colon wash-outs with aqueous enemas to promote evacuation, lead to conditions which are identical to those obtained with continuous perfusion: a colon which receives 6 or more liters of water in 24 hours, though maximizing its absorption of water and sodium, releases huge amounts of potassium, with consequences at general and local level. Cases have been observed of potassium depletion due to an excessive amount of enemas, showing symptoms such as nervous and cardiocirculatory failure and an atonic large intestine. Thus, a significant amount of motor neuroses of the colon demonstrated by X-ray examination do not show signs of a real functional pathology, but are secondary to the above mentioned hydroelectric alterations induced by the preparation phase to DCBE examination.

Therefore, radiologists should be advised to develop colon preparation protocols with no heavy impact on the absorption and excretion functions of the large intestine.

Secretion

The substances secreted by the colon include: *mucus*, with alkaline pH and high buffer property (1 mL:0.5 mL of HCl N10), mainly consisting of acid polysaccharides; *proteins*, the same found in the blood, and especially alpha and beta globulines [9]; *enzymes*, such as amylase and lysozyme. Most of the other enzymes commonly found in the feces, i.e. invertase, peptidase, proteinase and lipase, often come from the upper intestinal tract.

A normal individual forms about 1 L of a viscous and extremely water-rich secretion daily. Colon secretion has mainly a protective, mechanical and chemical function. The lubrication function of the feces and the colonic walls is self-evident, in order to facilitate stool progression and expulsion. With its pH (about 8), some products of bacterial fermentation are neutralized. Under the protective mucus layer, mucosa desquamation and regeneration go on undisturbed without any traumas which would otherwise occur if it were in direct contact with the feces.

Mucus secretion in the colon is thought to be regulated by the autonomic nervous system, by the mechanic action of the feces against the colonic wall as well as by "surface irritation factors" which give origin to a local-allergic type of reaction.

Under normal conditions, the large intestine mucus secretion is basically controlled by the autonomic nervous system (no hormonal influence has so far been observed). Stimulation of the parasympathetic system has been demonstrated to enhance the activity of goblet cells, whereas their function is inhibited by the sympathetic system [10]. Therefore, acetylcholine serves as neurotransmitter at the neuroglandular synapses. However, under experimental conditions, mucus secretion is enhanced also by other parasympathetic-cholinomimetic alkaloids, like pilocarpine and arecoline. Therefore, an antagonistic action is exerted between the sympathetic and parasympathetic system that, depending on which of them is prevailing, leads to deep changes in the amount of mucus in colon and feces.

Table 4. Secretion (enzymes, mucus, proteins)

- Colon secretion is subject to autonomic nervous system regulation and is under the action of a local mechanic system

- Secretion can be directly stimulated through a physical (high temperature, micro-traumas) or chemical (laxatives, irrigations, enemas) mechanism

In addition to nervous stimulation, the colon secretory activity can normally be stimulated also by other factors. Among them, mechanic irritation seems to be the most important one, caused by the intestinal mucosa rubbing against itself and the fecal mass, which is what happens during standard colon movements.

Finally, mucus secretion can be caused by a whole set of surface irritants which, when in contact with the mucosa, trigger an abundant myxorrhea, through an allergic type reaction.

From the above mentioned data, which are briefly illustrated in Table 4, it is clear that, with the indiscriminate use of enemas and peroral washouts, the colon secretory function is significantly altered, under the abnormal stimulation through physical or chemical contact with the administered substances which in turn lead to hypermyxorrhea.

This is often the cause of otherwise unexplainable diagnostic errors. Many situations labelled as "colon secretory neurosis" often fail to present real hypersecretory conditions, since they are due to the irritation on the bowel walls during DCBE preparatory phase.

The problem seems of difficult solution: the colon secretory function is not only affected by physicochemical agents, since it is also under the regulatory control of the sympathetic and parasympathetic systems. The development of a new preparation protocol for this examination, without enemas and drugs stimulating or inhibiting the autonomic nervous system, is therefore desirable.

Intestinal flora activity

The role of intestinal bacteria has been clearly explained in the last few decades with germ-free animals and suitable techniques [11,12]. The knowledge of the physiologic mechanisms by which the intestinal flora affects intestinal gas formation is very important for the radiologist.

Under physiologic conditions, significant amounts of gas are contained in the colon and minimum amounts in the small intestine. The global gas volume, deriving from ingested air, is about 1.3 L in the male and 0.6 L in the female. CO_2 accounts for 40%, N_2 for 50%, methane, hydrogen, hydrogen sulfide and fermentation products are also present. Gas is eliminated through the anus to a minimum extent (380-655 mL/day), while most of it is absorbed by the intestinal wall [13].

Intestinal gases originate through three different peculiar mechanisms: air ingested through swallowing, chemical production during digestion, and absorption through the blood flow. Therefore, meteorism can be due to excessive ingestion of air, excessive production of intestinal gases, and insufficient gas reabsorption.

In a single meal, up to 500 mL of air can be swallowed [14]. Excessive amounts of air are generally swallowed by heavy eaters or by particularly anxious or irritable people. In these latter type of "air eaters", in addition to increased breathing, hypersalivation is also developed by the autonomic nervous system.

Excessive air production in the intestine is often due to a hyper-fermentation of cellulose components contained in the food and to protein putrefaction following an unbalanced situation among in-

testinal contents, intestinal flora, digestion enzymes and bowel motility [15]. A slowing down in intestinal transit increases the digestive action of the intestinal flora in the colon, through which more gas is generated: the more digestion takes place in the colon, the greater is the amount of gas produced.

Gastric hyperacidity can be another, not so uncommon, cause of excessive gas production. The intestinal microbial balance is altered with subsequent protein hyperputrefaction, and hence gas production [16]. Also, conditions of impaired digestion are another cause of meteorism, whereby, due to a lack of digestion enzymes, excessive amounts of ingested food reach the colon [17]. Malabsorption caused by pancreatic insufficiency (chronic pancreatitis) is also important, as well as meteorism due to biliary diseases and mono- and polysaccharide maldigestion (maltase, isomaltase or other disaccharide deficiency).

As mentioned above, meteorism is also due to reduced gas reabsorption. This physiopathologic condition can occur in case of intestinal hypotonia with decreased intraluminal pressure [16]. Poor reabsorption is also present in case of venous congestion and ischemic colitis when the blood flow is unable to absorb and take away the produced gas [18].

Last but not least, occlusive and sub-occlusive conditions are another important cause of meteorism: in these cases, meteorism is caused by the fact that gases cannot move down to the anal sphincter for expulsion.

From the above explanation, two important considerations can be made for the radiologist:
1. enemas during preparation for DCBE upset the microbial flora in the colon so as to alter the physiologic mechanisms for air production;
2. the physical contact between the colonic mucosa and the introduced fluid reduces the amount of air physiologically absorbed by the colonic wall.

For this reason, the radiologist who during an examination observes an excessive amount of gas, must be very careful in formulating a "meteorism" diagnosis, without previously considering a whole series of potentially affecting factors, such as antibiotic therapy and the use of enemas and laxatives.

Motor activity

From a mechanical point of view, the colon serves for storage, transport and removal of intraluminal contents. These functions are made possible by the tonic and phasic motor activity of the intestinal walls. The most important colon movements are: segmentation, peristalsis, mass peristalsis, and adaptive relaxation.

Segmentation features contractions of the circular muscle forming pleats or sacculations (haustra). By mixing the intraluminal contents, this activity aims at favoring the absorption and secretion by the intestine, which mainly occurs in the transverse colon and in the descending and sigmoid colon.

Peristalsis consists of a coordinated movement characterized by a contraction wave preceded by a release wave which propels forward the colonic contents [19]. Though peristaltic movements are observed in all colon segments, they are rather infrequent and fecal progress through the large intestine does not seem to be directly determined by this type of motor activity.

The forward movement of the fecal mass is due to the so called *mass peristalsis*: a broad motion characterized by a propulsive contraction with subsequent pressure increase in the upstream colon segment associated with a muscle release in the downstream segment, where the haustral segmentation is obliterated, with subsequent pressure drop [20]. In this way, a high pressure gradient is formed between the two contiguous intestinal areas with subsequent forward propulsion of the colonic contents from the area having the higher pressure to the one with the lower pressure [21].

Adaptive relaxation is the property by which the colon adapts itself to progressively accommodate increasing fecal volumes without leading to intraluminal pressure increase, nor receptor stimulation due to intraparietal stretching. It is mainly characteristic of the cecum and the rectal ampulla.

Two fundamental laws regulating large bowel motility should be mentioned: Connell's law [22], and the pressure gradient law.

Connell's law, also called "Law of false constipation and/or paradoxical diarrhea" is based on the assumption that the more the colon is hyperkinetic (spastic), i.e. characterized by increased segmentation, the less propulsion activity will be. Viceversa, the more the colon is hypokinetic (atonic), i.e. characterized by reduced segmentation, the more propulsion activity will be.

Therefore, a constipated patient often has a hyperkinetic colon, whereas a hypokinetic or even atonic colon may be the expression of a functional diarrheal

syndrome. Hence, there is no direct proportional correlation between colon motor activity and the transit of the fecal mass, which is actually determined by proper integration of all the colonic movements causing adequate pressure gradients in the bowel.

According to the *pressure gradient law*, there is a mechanic gradient between the proximal and the distal colon and between the latter and the rectum, whereby, under normal conditions, colonic contents are prevented from moving from the right (low pressure) to the left (high pressure), while their transfer is favored from the sigmoid to the rectum. After meals, the gradient between the proximal and distal colon is reduced down to opposite values, namely with higher pressure on the right and lower pressure on the left.

What has been illustrated so far is important for the radiologist, particularly in the light of two precise objectives: to sort out the confusion in the classification adopted to define the various types of motor neurosis, and to allow a clear and informed comparison between the patient symptoms and the X-ray findings. For example, when a *spastic colon* is reported, an increase in segmentation activity and a reduction in propulsion movements must always be observed. Conversely, a report of *atonic colon* should be proved by a reduction or disappearance in segmentation and increase in propulsion. Finally, from a clinical point of view, most cases of constipation are characterized by colon hypersegmentation, whereas diarrheal syndromes are likely to be supported by an atonic bowel.

References

1. Levitan R, Fordtran JS, Burrows BA et al (1962) Isotonic saline composition; water and salt absorption in the human colon. J Clin Invest 41:1754
2. Davenport HW (1966) Physiology of the digestive tract. Chicago: Year Book Med Publ Inc
3. Devroede GJ, Phillips SF (1969) Conservation of sodium chloride and water by the human colon. Gastroenterology 56:101-109
4. Phillips SF, Giller G (1973) The contribution of the colon to electrolyte and water conservation in man. J Lab Clin Med 81:733-746
5. Foster EA, Sandle G, Hayslett JP et al (1981) Chronic potassium loading and cyclic AMP stimulate active potassium secretion in the rat colon. Gut 11:A893
6. Bernier JJ (1987) Trattato di Gastroenterologia. Roma: Delfino, Vol III, pp 1177-1191
7. Schields R, Miles JB (1965) Absorption and secretion in the large intestine. Postgrad Med J 41:435

8. Debongnie JC, Phillips SF (1978) Capacity of the human colon to absorb fluid. Gastroenterology 74:698-703

9. Soergel KH, Ingelfinger FJ (1964) Composition of rectal mucus in normal subjects and patients with ulcerative colitis. Gastroenterology 47:610-616

10. Gregory RA (1950) Some factor influencing the passage of fluid through intestinal loops in dogs. J Physiol 111:119

11. Gorbach SL (1971) Intestinal microflora. Gastroenterology 60:1110-1129

12. Drasar BS, Hill MJ (1974) Human intestinal flora. London: Academic Press, Vol I

13. Stocchi F (1961) Il meteorismo. Policlinico Prat 68:861-878

14. McNelly EF, Kelly JE, Ingelfinger FJ (1964) Mechanism of belching: effect of gastric distension with air. Gastroenterology 46:254-259

15. De Braych L, Veine S, Laurre M (1962) Les gas abdominaux et les meteorismes. Sem Hop Paris 38:2657-2666

16. Monges H, Vignoli R, Legre H (1971) Meteorisme. Paris: EMC

17. Kirk E (1949) La quantitè et la composition des gas coletiques. Gastroenterology 12:792-794

18. Chenf P, Desprez-Curely (1956) Les ballonements abdominaux. Gaz Med Fr 63:717-727

19. Bayliss M, Starling EH (1900) The movements and innervation of the large intestine. Br J Radiol 8:652

20. Holdstock DJ, Misiewicz JJ, Smith T et al (1970) Factors controlling motility: colonic pressures and transit after meals in patient with total gastrectomy, pernicious anemia or duodenal ulcer. Gut 11:100

21. Berti Riboli E, Reboa G, Frascio M (1994) Patologia funzionale in coloproctologia: Diagnosi, Terapia, Riabilitazione. Padova: Piccin, P 158-160

22. Connell AM (1962) The motility of the pelvic colon. II. Paradoxical motility in diarrhoea and constipation. Gut 3:342-348

7 Is diet control a compulsory step in the preparation to DCBE?

As effectively pointed out by Miller [1], a colon report must read either positive or negative, or it must be repeated. In this context, a thorough cleansing of the large bowel from any fecal contents is an absolutely essential pre-condition [2]. This will ensure against:

- incorrect X-ray diagnosis with significant increase in false negatives and false positives;
- need to repeat the examination;
- the troubles for the patient of a second examination and above all another, not negligible, radiation dose;
- excessive workload for the staff involved in the examination;
- extra costs for the community.

The cleansing of the large intestine is mainly obtained through the following three operations: a) *suitable diet in the days preceding the examination*; b) *laxatives*; and c) *cleansing enemas*. In this chapter the diet role will be discussed, from a theoretical and experimental point of view. Although opinions on dietary restrictions vary widely, the importance attributed to them is proved by the fact than only a small percentage among major institutions are not using any diet regime, while 9 out of 10 require a specific diet from their patients for 18-48 hours before the examination [3]. It should be noted that the "diet aspect" cannot be separated from the "type of laxative treatment", since, obviously enough, the effect required from the latter is dependent on the quantity and quality of ingested food.

As to *quantity*, the amount of ingested food is in most cases reduced (low amount of solid food, low-residue diet, liquid-only diet, starvation), though this reduction tends to slow down the transit of intestinal contents. With regard to the *quality* of ingested food, its plasticity is increased to allow for an easier expulsion of fecal material.

These apparently simple concepts have led to a two-fold result:

1. Poor attention to the need to prescribe a concrete and accurate diet. In the majority of cases, only empirical, very general and often superficial recommendations are made, which, in any case, are insufficient to properly prepare the patient. For example, at least 2 out of 3 patients when advised to follow "a low-residue diet" do not know exactly what they actually have to eat or not. Furthermore, whatever the diet, compliance is likely to be poorer without accurate instructions. From this point of view, some advantages are offered by pre-packaged low-residue [4] or liquid [5] diets.

2. A wrong assessment of the possible use of some beneficial properties of vegetable fibers, which play an important role in forming the fecal mass, namely its qualitative features, speed of intestinal transit and pressure levels inside the large intestine [6] (Fig. 1).

These two aspects, i.e. low-residue fiber-free diet or dietary fibers, were investigated by our group in Genoa already at the end of the '70s [7].

It should be noted here that the prescription by some Authors [8] of total fastening, except for liquids, in the days preceding the examination, cannot be supported from a physiopathologic point of view (compensatory secretion by the large intestine), nor from a correct practice rationale. The patient in most cases has to undergo several examinations within a brief period of time, all of them requiring absolute intestinal cleansing; therefore his/her compliance is very low to preparation protocols requiring a more or less long fastening period.

Low-residue fiber-free diet

The diet regimen developed by our institution (Tables 1 and 2) has a medium caloric value (2000 kcal), a balanced composition, a very low vegetable fiber content (2.26 g), and is abundant in liquids, specially during the day before the examination. The increased liquid intake compensates for the loss in fecal softness due to the fiber-free diet and minimizes the dehydration induced by laxatives.

Table 1. Low-residue fiber-free diet to be followed 3 and 2 days before DCBE examination

8 a.m.	a cup of partially skimmed milk; 4-6 slices of melba toast
10 a.m.	a glass of fruit juice
1 p.m.	40 g of pasta dressed with a tablespoon of olive oil; 100 g of lean beef hamburger grilled or steamed; one boiled or mashed potato; 40 g of non-fat cheese; 25 g of fat-free bread sticks; a jar of baby-food fruit; a glass of fruit juice
4 p.m.	a glass of fruit juice
8 p.m.	20 g of pasta dressed with a tablespoon of olive oil; 150 g of lean fish or 100 g of beef as above; one boiled or mashed potato; 40 g of non-fat cheese; 25 g of fat-free bread sticks; a jar of baby-food fruit
	During the day, drink at least 2 liters of liquid: i.e. non-carbonated water, coffee, tea, camomile tea, lean vegetable or beef broth
	Sugar, alcoholic beverages and carbonated water are not permitted

	LOW FIBER AMOUNT	HIGH FIBER AMOUNT
FECAL MASS		
TRANSIT TIME		
INTESTINAL PRESSURE		
BACTERIAL FLORA		

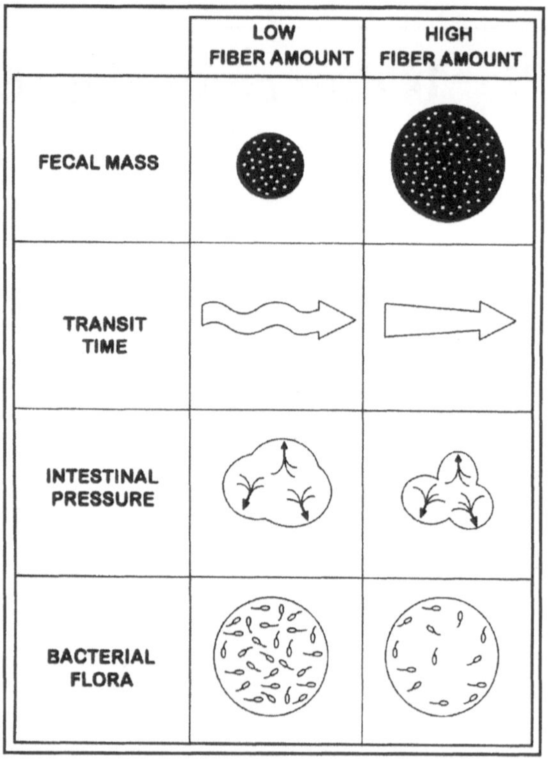

Fig. 1. Some beneficial properties of vegetable fibers

Table 2. Diet regimen to be followed the day before DCBE examination

8 a.m.	a small yogurt or a cup of partially skimmed milk
1 p.m.	70 g of small pasta dressed with a tablespoon of olive oil and grated Parmesan cheese; 150 g of lean beef hamburger grilled or steamed without fats
8 p.m.	a cup of lean beef or vegetable broth
	Sugar, alcoholic beverages and carbonated water are not permitted

In order to achieve an actual change in the quality and quantity of fecal material, the proposed diet has to start at least three days before the examination. This is not particularly suitable for urgent cases. Nevertheless, only a slight difference in the results is observed in case of a forced reduction in the preparation period [9].

Based on the large experience acquired, we are able to maintain the cleansing of the large intestine, obtained by matching this diet regimen with cathartic sennosides/$MgSO_4$ treatment, absolutely satisfactory. It should be stressed once again that the use of cleansing enemas is unnecessary. Changes in the diet required for therapeutical reasons (diverticulosis and its complications, irritable bowel syndrome, chronic constipation), whereby the diet is enriched with high-residue fibers, may actually be a weakness of this method.

Properties of dietary fiber

Dietary fiber, the indigestible natural packing of plant foods, is a combination of a heterogeneous group of substances, most notably cellulose, hemicellulose and lignin. Physicochemical properties differ among the various types of plants and, within the same type, depend on its growth and maturation conditions. Their major properties are:

- *water-holding capacity*. It varies significantly depending on the type of fiber and above all on polysaccharide contents. Withheld water, which is partly adsorbed and partly distributed in the intermolecular space of polysaccharides, serves as "ballast" in the large intestine, by increasing the bulk and softness of feces.
- *biliary acid absorption*. This is a direct function in the intestine. The removal of biliary acids from the entero-hepatic circulation reduces the uptake of exogenous fatty acids and cholesterol.
- *electrolytic exchange*. There is a good correlation between fiber hydrophilic properties and ion exchange. However, the range of such effect depends on the type of fiber: some increase sodium, others potassium, magnesium, phosphorus and iron excretion. More variable results are obtained with regard to calcium.

Dietary fiber has favorable effects on intestinal mucosae through an increase in enzyme and hormone secretion and motility, due to longer mastication required and greater food volume, and also through the reduction in water absorption by the intestinal mucosa with subsequent increase in the bulk, softness and lubrication of stool.

The total fiber intake ranges between 4 and 10 g per day and up to 12-24 g in vegetarian diets. The type of diet adopted by technologically and socially advanced populations plays a major role in the onset of several colon diseases. The use of more refined foods, thus with a lower amount of residues,

undoubtedly promotes the onset of lesions in the colon and rectum, specially in more susceptible and sensitized individuals. Therefore, vegetable fiber in the diet, that is not digested by human enzymes in the small intestine but undergoes only partial hydrolysis by the local bacterial and fungal flora, protects against the onset of many colon diseases. Figure 2 illustrates the pathogenic mechanisms likely to lead to colon disturbances due to fiber-poor diets [10].

Dietary fiber

A sudden change in the diet is likely to provoke temporary changes in colon functions until it adapts to the new condition. Also, most people affected by overt colon diseases are already following a targeted high-residue diet for therapeutical reasons. Therefore, we thought it advisable to assess the colon cleansing level of patients prepared to the DCBE with a fiber-rich diet. From certain aspects, when looking at their properties, vegetable fibers can be considered to be beneficial to a good intestinal cleansing. They indeed act as a large broom capable of picking up all residues in the intestinal lumen, thus making feces more compact and easier to be expelled.

To what extent, then, is a sudden reduction in fiber content in the diet an advantage for these patients (due to the expected better cleansing of the large bowel [11-14])? And when, conversely, is it rather a disadvantage (due to induced secondary functional reactions)? This aspect is important especially if we consider how often the question of irritable bowel syndrome is raised, particularly in referral centers. These patients should be prepared for the DCBE with the utmost respect for their basic functional condition, also with regard to their usual diet.

The diet regimen presented in Table 3 has been tested on 40 patients specifically referred for a DCBE. At the end of the second day of diet the usual cathartic sennosides/$MgSO_4$ treatment was administered, as already described in Chapter 4. The results obtained have been assessed on the radiographs made during the DCBE examination. Cleansing level received different scores: from *excellent* (total absence of fecal residues), *good* (minimum fecal residues which would not hamper a fine analysis of the colonic mucosa), *fair* (noticeable fe-

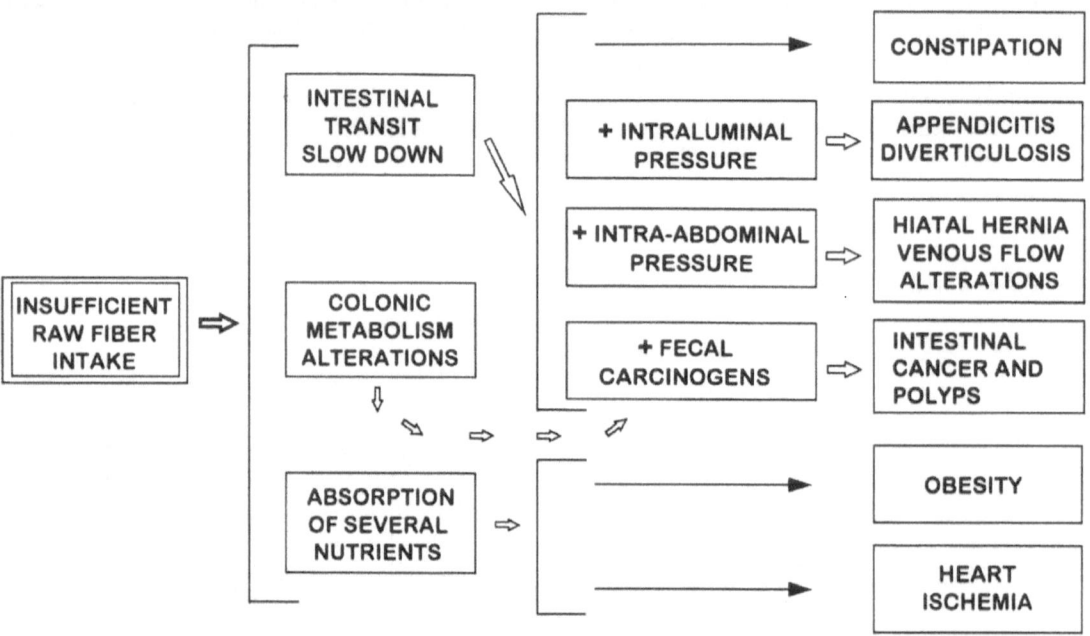

Fig. 2. Pathogenic mechanisms leading to colon disturbances due to customary insufficient raw fiber intake

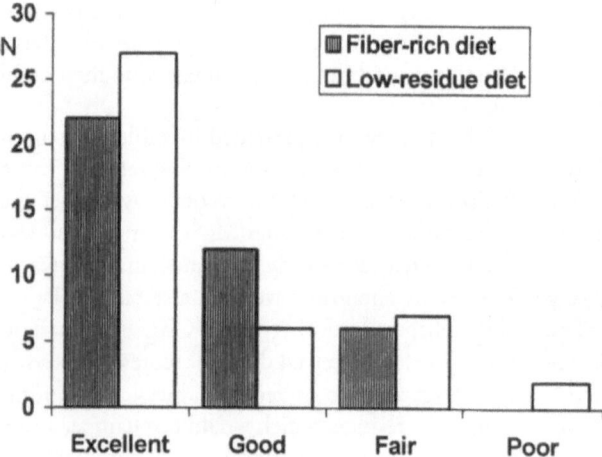

Fig. 3. Colon cleansing levels of patients prepared to DCBE with fiber-rich diet or low-residue diet

cal residues which would not hamper an accurate diagnostic evaluation), and *poor* (considerable fecal residues requiring a re-examination). The results are fully comparable with those obtained in other 42 patients prepared in a similar way but on a low-residue diet (Fig. 3).

Table 3. High-residue fiber-rich diet to be followed 3 and 2 days before DCBE examination

8 a.m.	a small yogurt or half a cup of partially skimmed milk; two tablespoons of bran; 2-4 slices of whole-wheat melba toast; a tablespoon of honey
1 p.m.	100 g of whole-wheat pasta with tomato sauce and a tablespoon of olive oil and grated Parmesan cheese; 100 g lean beef hamburger grilled or steamed; mixed salad dressed with a tablespoon of olive oil; 50 g of non-fat cheese; 3-6 slices of whole-wheat melba toast; either an apple, a pear, an orange or prunes
4 p.m.	either an apple, a pear or cooked prunes without sugar
8 p.m.	2 tablespoons of small whole-wheat pasta in broth with grated Parmesan cheese; 150 g of lean fish or meat grilled or steamed; cooked vegetables dressed with a tablespoon of olive oil; 3-6 slices of whole-wheat melba toast; either an apple, a pear, an orange or prunes
	During the day, at least 2 liters of liquid: i.e. noncarbonated water, coffee, tea, camomile tea, lean vegetable or beef broth
	Sugar, alcoholic beverages and carbonated water are not permitted

More recently, also Hellström and Brolin [15] and Fork [16] have obtained the same results. In particular, the former ones maintain that the discontinuation of an earlier instituted dietary fiber medication before a barium enema does not seem justified since dietary fiber does not have a negative effect on colon cleansing, but may instead have a beneficial effect, which is possibly more pronounced in patients with constipation.

Our direct experience induces us to accept the following conclusions:

- the cathartic treatment used at the end of the controlled diet strongly affects the various results obtained with different diets: with the sennosides/$MgSO_4$ association, these effects are certainly minimized;
- if this type of cathartic treatment is adopted, either of the two diet regimens can be selected irrespective of their residue content;
- in practice, either of the two can be used if so required for therapeutical reasons by the basal colon disease in a specific patient. By doing so, there will be less problems involved in a sudden change of diet as well as risks of provoked and non-spontaneous functional reactions;
- the choice of a free diet regimen seems to us less easy to be supported since, by doing so, the theoretical assumptions favoring the use of a fiber-free or a fiber-rich diet would no longer apply;
- in no case can proper patient hyperhydration be neglected, also and above all, as we shall see, to ensure against the negative effects on the mucosal coating induced by the absorption of water by the colonic mucosa from the barium suspension.

References

1. Miller RE (1976) The clean colon. Gastroenterology 70:289-290
2. Eyler W (1969) In: Detection of colon lesions, First Standardization Conference. Chicago, American College of Radiology, 1973. p 108
3. Thoeni RF, Margulis AR (1988) The state of radiographic technique in the examination of the colon: A survey in 1987. Radiology 167:7-12
4. Gutwein I, Baer J, Holt PR (1981) The effect of a formula diet on preparation of the colon for barium enema examination: Impact on health care and costs. Arch Intern Med 141:993-996
5. Tham RTOTA, Korte JH, Bom EP et al (1993) Preparation of the colon for single- and double-contrast barium enema examination: A simplified method. Radiology, 188:578-580
6. Cairella M, Godi R. La fibra alimentare. Roma: Società Editrice Universo, 1978.
7. Oliva L, Cittadini G (1981) Il clisma a doppio contrasto: problemi metodologici e tecnici. Verona: Cortina, pp 71-77
8. De Lacey G, Benson M, Wilkins R et al (1982) Routine colonic lavage is unnecessary for double-contrast barium enema in outpatients. BMJ 284:1021-1022
9. Kember PG, McBride KD, Tweed CS, Collins MC (1995)

A blinded prospective trial of low-residue versus normal diet in preparation for barium enema. Br J Radiol 68:128-129

10. Trowell HC, Burkitt DP (1975) Refined carbohydrate foods and disease: Some implications of dietary fibre. London: Academic Press

11. Kendrick RGM, MacKenzie S, Beckly DE (1981) A comparison of four methods of bowel preparation for barium enema. Clin Radiol 32:95-97

12. Virkki R, Mäkelä P (1983) Low residual diet and hydration improving double contrast examination of the colon. Eur J Radiol 3:212-214

13. Lee JR, Ferrando JR (1984) Variables in the preparation of the large intestine for double contrast barium enema examination. Gut 25:69-72

14. Gelfand DW, Chen MYM, Ott DJ (1991) Preparing the colon for the barium enema examination. Radiology 178:609-613

15. Hellström M, Brolin I (1987) Dietary fibers in the preparation of the bowel for diagnostic barium enema. Gastrointest Radiol 12:76-78

16. Fork FT (1988) Wheat fibre before radiography of the large bowel. Acta Radiol 29:375

8 Cathartics and their combination

By cathartic we mean any substance which, administered orally or, less commonly, in other ways, promotes or accelerates the emptying of the large intestine or of both the small and large intestines.

Depending on the induced effect, cathartics are divided into *laxatives* (suitable for a regular use in some forms of constipation), *purgatives* (suitable for occasional use) and *drastics* (almost abandoned, because of their excessively intensive effect). However, this intensity, which is partially affected by individual tolerance, mainly depends on the administered dosage: almost all cathartics can have the above three effects, by progressively increasing the dose.

In several X-ray examinations, the intestinal lumen has to be cleansed of food and fecal contents, which can be done through a rational use of purgative cathartics. An ideal purgative must have the following features:
- no toxicity;
- no interference with digestion;
- no interference with the absorption of nutrients: on this point, the time of administration of the purgative is extremely important;
- no induction of excessive loss of endogenous water, which in any case can be minimized through concurrent patient hyperhydration;
- no significant interference with the hydrosaline balance, specially with regard to purgatives that act through an anti-absorption mechanism;
- possibility to achieve consistent and repeatable effects;
- acceptable taste without unpleasant aftertaste;
- sufficient effect to avoid the use of cleansing enemas.

The cleansing of the intestinal lumen is understandably paramount in the preparation to the DCBE, for which *individual purgatives* or *combinations of purgatives* have repeatedly been tested, with or without cleansing enemas.

Since it is the radiologist who is responsible for the examination and its either positive or negative report, he/she has to exert great care in selecting and prescribing the right bowel preparation [1,2]. For this purpose, an adequate knowledge of individual purgatives is essential, with regard to their cathartic effects as well as to any side effects, risks and contraindications to their use.

A simple classification of purgatives is based on their mechanisms of action (Table 1). Due to their large use in bowel preparation of patients before DCBE, *saline* and *irritant* purgatives will be considered here, making reference to the characteristics affecting the way they are employed [3].

Table 1. Classification of purgatives according to mechanisms of action

1.	Agents to increase the bulk of intestinal contents osmotic salines hydrophilic colloidals
2.	Lubricant purgatives emollients/lubricants tensioactives
3.	Irritant purgatives irritants proper contact laxatives

Saline purgatives

These purgatives act by inducing an osmotic flow of water toward the intestinal lumen. The most commonly used are: **magnesium sulfate** (or Epsom salt), $MgSO_4 \cdot 7H_2O$; **sodium sulfate** (or Glauber salt), $Na_2SO_4 \cdot 10H_2O$; **magnesium citrate**, $Mg_3(C_6H_5O_7)_2 \cdot H_2O$.

Their action mechanism is based on the fact that Mg^{++}, SO_4^{--} and $C_6H_5O_7^{---}$ ions are poorly absorbed by the intestinal mucosa, that acts as a semipermeable membrane separating the plasmatic compartment from the intestinal content [3]. When the salt is administered in hypertonic solution, it draws fluid in the intestinal lumen until an isotonic condition is reached. Such isotonic condition with the body fluids is achieved with a 4% and 3.2% magnesium sulfate and sodium sulfate concentration, respectively. When administered in the usual purgative dose of 15 g, they draw - assuming that the salt is not reabsorbed - 400 and 500 mL of water, respectively, in the intestinal tract. This amount of fluids is enough to stimulate pressoreceptors along the whole intestine, thus inducing peristaltic rushes. To ensure the patient against dehydration, it is sufficient for him/her to drink 1.5-2 L of water over the 2-3 hours since administration of the saline purgative.

The action of saline purgatives is very fast: it starts after about thirty minutes and is over around three hours after intake. **Sodium sulfate** is slightly more effective than **magnesium sulfate** but has a bad taste. **Magnesium citrate** used as a flavored water solution, which the addition of sodium bicarbonate and citric acid makes effervescent, though with a pleasant taste has quite a mild effect. The usual dose is 25 g of salt dissolved in 250 mL of water.

The risks involved in the use of Mg^{++} salts in patients with chronic renal failure have been stressed by several Authors [2,4,5]. These patients have difficulties in eliminating the absorbed magnesium fraction (which may reach up to 20-40%), with subsequent build-up of extracellular fluids. In our more than 20 years experience, the routine use of magnesium sulfate, which is a cheap drug with a constant and well controllable effect, has never led to any, not even minor side effect. However, generally speaking, every saline purgative may be contraindicated in subjects with congestive heart failure and should be administered only to those with good renal functions.

Saline purgatives interact with the small intestine: intestinal contents remain fluid, rapidly flow through the large intestine and are then expelled. There are good reasons to believe that an unpredictable amount of salt is likely to remain in the large intestine for a more or less long period of time, thus interacting with the barium suspension during DCBE implementation, by absorbing free water from the suspension (see Chapter 15). For this reason, the barium suspension concentration has to be modified when saline purgatives are used for bowel preparation.

Mannitol, a straight-chain alcohol with six hydroxyl groups, has no direct action on the bowel, is poorly absorbed and retains fluid within the lumen by osmosis, distending the intestine and thereby inducing intestinal hurry. Administered in a 200 g dose, it is slowly ingested dissolved in 1-2 liters of water. This mildly effective purgative was first proposed for intestinal preparation to DCBE in 1979 [6]. However, after doubts were raised about its use [7], and modifications proposed to its dose, timing and sequence [8], it was finally suggested to abandon it [9].

Irritant purgatives

We shall consider: **castor oil**, the conventional reference purgative, **contact laxatives**, very popular in the United States, **anthraquinonic derivatives**, which, for reasons we are going to explain below, are those preferred in the Genoa technique.

Castor oil is a triglyceride ricinoleic acid. In the small intestine, after hydrolysis by pancreatic lipase, it is turned into glycerin and ricinoleic acid - the real active principle which also has a remarkable irritant action on the mucosa of the small intestine and an anti-absorption effect with respect to sodium and water. It has no effect in the large intestine since ricinoleic acid, like all dietary fats, after its total absorption by the small intestine, enters the body circulation. Any fraction of castor oil eventually reaching the large intestine will be inactive, since, lacking any lipolytic enzymes, it will not be split. As a result, only little intestinal griping is associated with the action of castor oil.

Castor oil is particularly beneficial in those cases where the use of purgatives with a direct effect on the large intestine would be dangerous because of an ongoing colon inflammation. The purgative dose is 40-60 mL: 1-2 semiliquid discharges are obtained after 2-6 hours. Stool is watery because of the rapid flow of the chyme through the small intestine, thus preventing normal water absorption. Glycerin released by enzymatic hydrolysis becomes a lubricant as well as an irritant to the intestinal mucosa with capillary dilation and increase in mucus secretion. The particularly unpleasant taste of castor oil can be partially disguised by mixing it with a suitable amount of sweetened milk. Since castor oil has no effect on the large intestine, in the preparation to DCBE it must always be used in association with cleansing enemas.

In 50% of patients taking castor oil only once for purgative purposes, giant multinucleated cells are found in the urine from 12 to 25 hours after intake [10]. There is no clear physiopathologic explanation to this finding: however, the anti-absorption effect of castor oil in the small intestine is thought to be responsible for kidney overloading.

In 1962, the introduction in clinical practice of a few derivatives of biphenyl-piridyl-methane - bisacodyl in particular - drew the attention to the category of cathartics known as **contact laxatives**. The name refers to the fact that the action on the large intestine smooth muscles occurs after direct stimulation of the nervous plexuses of the mucosa in the region of contact, thus inducing parasympathetic reflexes that produce colonic peristaltic rushes without spasm. A concurrent anti-absorption mechanism may lead to the block of the sodium pump, complete calcium absorption inhibition by the colonic mucosa, and a conspicuous transfer of potassium from the intracellular space to the colonic lumen.

Bisacodyl (Dulcolax, Boehringer Ingelheim), administered orally in a 20 mg dose taken as four 5-mg tablets, has its effect after 6-12 hours. When administered through the rectum in a 10 mg dose, it has almost immediate effect. Abdominal cramps are an expected side effect. However, the effects are too often insufficient to meet the cleansing level needed for a DCBE examination. Therefore, it has to be associated with other purgatives (a popular association is with magnesium citrate) and with cleansing enemas. When taken in the usual dose, its action is limited to the large intestine.

Anthraquinonic purgatives (rhubarb, aloe, cascara and senna) act on the large intestine exclusively. Here, after minimum 6 hours since intake, effec-

tive peristaltic rushes are induced due to the stimulation of the Auerbach's myenteric plexus and, to a lower extent, through an irritant action on the mucosa.

Their active principles, emodins, are derivatives of anthraquinone which in turn is an anthracene compound. Cascara sagrada, used in the bowel preparation regimen suggested by Welin [11], as well as senna, have frangula emodin as active principle, which is partly free and partly bound to glucose in the form of inactive glucoside. After its absorption by the small intestine, this glucoside is hydrolyzed in the blood. Released emodin is eliminated through the large intestine where it exerts its effect. In routinary use as laxative, possible side effects are a brown coloration of the urine and melanosis coli.

Based on a long experience in the use of cascara and senna, we consider the latter substance to be much more effective in the emptying of the large intestine. The use of two purifiable and crystallizable glucosides (sennoside A and B) is particularly advantageous. It is indeed possible to grade their effect in a well reproducible form, thus overcoming all the problems connected with the use of senna extracts, whose inconsistent composition is likely to yield uncertain results.

After 6 hours from ingestion of a 150 mg mixture consisting of sennoside A and B calcium salts in equal parts, 1-2 solid discharges are induced, enough to empty the large intestine of its contents [12]. This gentle purgation rarely induces side-effects and spontaneous adverse comments by the patients. Since this effect is maintained for at least 6 hours, it is possible to induce the discharge of the small intestine later on when the large intestine is still "activated", thus achieving a complete cleansing of the digestive tract. The bowel preparation regimen for the DCBE now routinely performed at our institution is based on this approach. Intestinal cleansing without enemas is thus possible in a simple, innocuous and effective way (see Chapter 10).

Combinations of cathartics

We can say without exaggeration that there are as many protocols of intestinal preparation to the DCBE as the number of Authors who are specifically concerned with this examination. Almost all of them are based on a period of controlled diet, association of several purgatives, hyperhydration and sometimes cleansing enemas.

It should be pointed out that even the best bowel preparation for colonoscopy may not be so suitable for DCBE since, in the latter case, in addition to the cleansing of the intestinal lumen, attention must be paid not to interfere with the factors favoring an adequate mucosal coating [13].

In a general way, we agree with Miller [14] that "patient preference, although desirable, is not the prime factor in a cancer procedure". Nevertheless, an adequate bowel preparation often requires a balance between the desire to obtain a really clean colon and the distress caused to the patient [15]. Distress may be such as to require suspension of any working activity of the patient, need to stay close to a lavatory, interruption in night sleep, and, less commonly, the onset of real side effects, i.e. nausea, vomiting, feebleness, dizziness, headache, griping, cramping, abdominal pain.

It is not our intention to underestimate the value of many of the proposed intestinal preparation protocols, also because they may actually yield different results depending on how much conviction is placed in their implementation and on patient compliance. However, we shall examine those that have proved to be more effective and convenient, as demonstrated by the experience of those Authors who most of all have worked with the DCBE examination of the colon.

The **castor oil/cleansing enema combination** was the most popular bowel preparation regimen until the '70s, used as benchmark for new protocols [16]. A 60 mL dose of castor oil is ingested 16 hours before the examination. Thirteen and three hours before the examination, a cleansing enema is also performed. In controlled studies, the percentage of patients with a clean colon does not exceed 54-57%. The most controversial point in this protocol, for the reasons we shall see later on, is the need for cleansing enemas.

One of the regimens proposed by Welin [11], the latest and perhaps also the best thought-out, the **Cascara/Salax combination**, features 15 g of magnesium sulfate plus two 2 mg tablets of cascara sagrada, administered concurrently 24 and 18 hours before the examination. The cleansing enema is done only in patients with a particularly torpid intestine. According to the figures reported by the Author, a cleansed colon is achieved in 95% of patients. This association has given good results also in children, in which, when aged 6 to 10 years, the dosage is halved [17].

The bowel preparation regimen proposed by Brown [18], still very popular in the United States, is based on the **magnesium citrate/bisacodyl combination**. A 25 g dose of magnesium citrate is ingested in the afternoon preceding the examination. Then, five hours after the citrate, 20 mg of bisacodyl are administered orally and again in the morning of the examination in form of a 10 mg suppository. The saline produces a fluid bowel content which is readily evacuated under the action of the contact laxative drug. No subsequent investigators have been able to duplicate the claimed 95% of patients with thoroughly cleansed colon: the results vary between 32% [19] and 90% [20].

A **combination of magnesium citrate and sodium picosulfate**, a cathartic that like bisacodyl is hydrolyzed to hydroxyphenyl-pyridyl-methane [21], has gained consistent favour with British radiologists [22, 23]. The proprietary compound, Picolax (Ferring Pharmaceuticals, Middlesex), contains 13 g magnesium citrate and 10 mg sodium picosulfate in each of two sachets: one is taken mixed with water during the morning before the examination, the second eight hours later. The amount of thoroughly cleansed colon vary from 77% [24] to 95-96% [22, 25], but other experiences failed to prove any difference from the results obtained with magnesium citrate alone [26], with rapid oral colonic lavage solutions, or with cleansing enema alone [27]. There are important reports of side-effects related to sodium picosulfate - skin reactions, gastrointestinal disorders, headaches, hypoglycemia and one death from cardiac arrest [28, 29]. Therefore, this preparation regimen is still to be performed with the utmost caution.

A preparation regimen that has yielded very interesting results is the one proposed by Gelfand, Chen and Ott [30, 31], **the standard Bowman Gray preparation**. In the afternoon preceding the examination, 296 mL of a standard effervescent magnesium citrate solution are administered, followed 4 hours later by 59 mL of flavored castor oil. A cleansing enema consisting of 1,500 mL of warm tap water is administered the morning of the examination, and repeated once or twice if the returns are not clear. 97% of the barium enema examinations show good cleansing of the colon. The Authors absolutely insist on the importance of the cleansing enema.

In Italy, the preparation regimen according to **the Genoa protocol** is very popular [12]. It involves the administration of a saline purgative after colon activation with an anthraquinonic purgative. In this regimen, whose rational will be discussed in Chapter 10, no cleansing enema is required.

Oral colonic lavage solutions

An alternative way to the association of cathartics is the colonic lavage by rapid ingestion of a large volume of an iso-osmotic saline solution. After the first clinical trials of standard saline solutions, successful for what concerns intestinal cleansing, but engraved by a conspicuous absorption of water and sodium [32,33], an improved electrolyte solution was derived by substituting sodium sulfate for some of the sodium chloride and adding polyethylene glycol (PEG or macrogol 4000) to adjust osmolality (Golytely, Braintree Labs, Braintree, MA) [34]. Later on, a reduced sodium sulfate solution with increased PEG content was proposed [35].

Four liters of solution are administered orally in the afternoon preceding the examination [36-41]. The solution is not absorbed from the intestine and does not induce a loss of salt and water from the body. Fecal excretion results to be 94-100%. Golytely has been shown to be a safe, effective method of colon cleansing, and has become the preparation of choice for colonoscopy [42].

However, as above said, even the best bowel preparation for colonoscopy may not be so suitable for DCBE [13]. In fact, the results concerning the adecuacy of the oral lavage method for colon cleansing prior to barium enema are conflicting [13,42]. Though feces in the colon are generally less in the lavage than in the control groups, poor mucosal coating, due to excess fluid retained in the colon lumen, seems to be Golytely's greatest shortcoming as a barium enema preparation [37,38].

Administering Golytely during the middle of the day preceding the barium enema may reduce fluid retention within the colon [39]. Degraded mucosal coating may be corrected by the administration of bisacodyl just after [38,41] or before [40] Golytely ingestion.

Golytely can be used satisfactorily as an alternative to standard cathartics preparation especially in the elderly or debilitated patients or patients with hepatic, renal, or cardiac disease [39]. Side effects

of the preparation may limit its use as an outpatient preparation [41]. Unwillingness to use the preparation a second time was reported in a significant percentage of patients [41].

Many preparations belonging to the Golytely family have been tried in Europe (Colopeg, Oralav, Cololyt, Klean-Prep). In our department Isocolan (Bracco, Milan, Italy) was successfully tested in the preparation for barium enema of elderly and debilitated patients [43]. Selg (Promefarm, Milan, Italy) was largely used both alone as a rapid colonic lavage solution, and in association with sennosides [44].

Selg is an iso-osmotic saline preparation containing per liter: PEG 4000 58.30 g; Na_2SO_4 5.68 g; $NaHCO_3$ 1.68 g; NaCl 1.46 g; KCl 0.74 g; sodium cyclamate, acesulfame K, sodium saccharine, natural flavoring, maltodextrin, as excipients. With this formulation water and sodium absorption by the small intestine is blocked, while intraluminal contents are maintained iso-osmotic to extracellular spaces. Hence, the volume of fluid flowing into the colon is such that it saturates bowels absorption capacity and causes a watery asymptomatic diarrhea, which increases progressively with ingested volume increase. The addition of simethicone (0.08 g per liter) makes the Selg-Esse formulation different from the previous one. Simethicone's main physicochemical properties are: to reduce surface tension and allow the gas bubbles in the gastrointestinal tract to pool together and form free gas that is easily discharged; as a result, mucosal details are better visible at colonoscopy [45].

The toxicologic profile of both formulations with regard to the epithelium and colonic mucosa goblet cells is very favorable if compared with cathartic preparations containing magnesium citrate or sennosides [45].

The positive results we obtained with Selg are referred to in Chapter 10.

References

1. Miller RE (1978) The clean colon: whose responsibility? AJR 131:182-183
2. Irwin JP, Peterson GH (1982) Colon preparation for the barium enema: A guide for the radiologist. Gastrointest Radiol 7:75-78
3. Goodman LS, Gilman A (1980) The pharmacological basis of therapeutics. 6th ed. New York: Macmillan. p 1002-1012
4. Rosengren JE, Aberg T (1975) Cleansing the colon without enemas. Radiologe 15:421-426

5. Gelfand DW, Chen MYM, Ott DJ (1991) Preparing the colon for the barium enema examination. Radiology 178:609-613

6. Palmer KR, Khan AN (1979) Oral mannitol: A simple and effective bowel preparation for barium enema. BMJ 2:1038

7. Lee JR, Hares MM, Keighley MRB (1981) A randomized trial to investigate X-Prep, oral mannitol, and colonic washout for double contrast barium enema. Clin Radiol 32:591-594

8. Foord KD (1982) Oral mannitol as a preparation for double contrast barium enema. Clin Radiol 33:467-469

9. Foord KD, Morcos SK, Ward P (1983). A comparison of mannitol and magnesium citrate preparations for double-contrast barium enema. Clin Radiol 34:309-312

10. MacFarlane EW (1966) The appearance of multinucleated cells in the urine after purgation. Acta Cytol 10:104-109

11. Welin S, Welin G (1976) The double contrast examination of the colon. Experience with the Welin modification. Stuttgart: Thieme pp 5-11

12. Oliva L, Cittadini G (1981) Il clisma a doppio contrasto: problemi metodologici e tecnici. Verona: Cortina

13. Bakran A, Bradley JA, Breshnihan E et al (1977) Whole gut irrigation: An inadequate preparation for double contrast barium enema examination. Gastroenterology 73:28-30

14. Miller RE (1976) The clean colon. Gastroenterology 70:289-290

15. Downing R, Dorricott NJ, Keighley MRB et al (1978) Modification of the physiological disturbance produced by whole gut irrigation by preliminary mannitol administration. Brit J Surg 65:827

16. Dodds WJ, Scanlon GT, Shaw DK et al (1977) An evaluation of colon cleansing regimens. AJR 128:57-59

17. Reither M (1980) Erfahrungen mit Cascara-Salax bei der vorbereitung von kindern zur kolonkontrastdarstellung. Roentgenbl 33: 418-421

18. Brown GR (1961) A new approach to colon preparation for barium enema: preliminary report. Univ Mich Med Bull 27:225-230

19. Benson M, Harper J. A comparative double-blind trial of mannitol and magnesium citrate/bisacodyl (MCB) in the preparation of barium enema patients. Australas Radiol 1983; 27:25-26

20. Shaw MRP, Tait KB (1983) A clinical comparison of bowel preparations prior to double contrast barium enema. Australas Radiol 27:254-257

21. Jauch R, Hankwitz R, Beschke K et al (1975) Bis-(p-hydroxyphenyl)-pyridyl-2-methane: the common laxative principle of bisacodyl and sodium picosulphate. Arzneimittelforschung 25:1896-1900

22. De Lacey G, Benson M, Wilkins R et al (1982) Routine colonic lavage is unnecessary for double contrast barium enemas in outpatients. BMJ 284:1021-1022

23. Lee JR, Ferrando JR. Variables in the preparation of the large intestine for double contrast barium enema examination. Gut 1984; 25:69-72

24. Swarbrick MJ, Collins MC, Moore DJ et al (1994) A comparative trial of magnesium citrate (Citramag) and Picolax for barium enema bowel preparation. Clin Radiol 49:379-381

25. Chakraverty S, Hughes T, Keir MJ et al (1994) Preparation of the colon for double-contrast barium enema: Comparison of Picolax, Picolax with cleansing enema and Citramag (2 sachets) - A randomized prospective trial. Clin Radiol 49:566-569

26. Lee JR (1984) Combinations of laxatives for bowel preparation: Are they necessary? Clin Radiol 35:461-462

27. Lai AKH, Kwok PCH, Man SW et al (1996) A blinded clinical trial comparing conventional cleansing enema, Pico-salax and Golytely for barium enema bowel preparation. Clin Radiol 51:566-569

28. McBride KD (1992) Sodium picosulphate: reaction or drug interaction? Clin Radiol 45:290

29. Lawrance JAL, Massoud TF, Creasy TS et al (1994) Colonic preparation with Picolax: patient tolerance and approaches to fluid replacement. Clin Radiol 49:35-37

30. Gelfand DW, Chen YM, Ott DJ (1988) Colonic cleansing for radiographic detection of neoplasia: Efficacy of the magnesium citrate-castor oil-cleansing enema regimen. AJR 151:705-708

31. Gelfand DW, Chen YM, Ott DJ (1991) Preparing the colon for the barium enema examination. Radiology 178:609-613

32. Hewitt J, Rigby J, Reeve J et al (1973) Whole-gut irrigation in preparation for large-bowel surgery. Surgery Lancet 2:337-340

33. Levy AG, Benson JW, Hewlett E et al (1976) Saline lavage: a rapid, effective and acceptable method for cleansing the gastrointestinal tract. Gastroenterology 70: 157-161

34. Davis GR, Santa Ana CA, Morawski SG et al (1980) Development of a lavage solution associated with minimal water and electrolyte absorption or secretion. Gastroenterology 78:991-995

35. Fordtran JS, Santa Ana CA, Cleveland MB. A low sodium solution for gastrointestinal lavage. Gastroenterology 1990; 98: 11-16

36. Ernstoff JJ, Howard DA, Marshall JB et al (1983) A randomized blinded clinical trial of a rapid colonic lavage solution (Golytely) compared with standard preparation for colonoscopy and barium enema. Gastroenterology 84:1512-1516

37. Davis GR, Smith HJ (1983) Double-contrast examination of the colon after preparation with Golytely (a balanced lavage solution). Gastrointest Radiol 8:173-176

38. Girard CM, Rugh KS, DiPalma JA et al (1984) Comparison of Golytely lavage with standard diet/cathartic preparation for double-contrast barium enema. AJR 142:1147-1149

39. Chan CH, Diner WC, Fontenot E et al. Randomized single-blind clinical trial of a rapid colonic lavage solution (Golytely) vs. standard preparation for barium enema and colonoscopy. Gastrointest Radiol 1985; 10:378-382

40. Fitzsimons P, Shorvon P, Frost RA et al (1987) A comparison of Golytely and standard preparation for barium enema. J Can Assoc Radiol 38:109-112

41. Tomlinson TL, DiPalma JA, Mangano FA. Comparison of a new colon lavage solution (Golytely-RSS) with a standard preparation for air-contrast barium enema. AJR 1988; 151:947-950

42. Thoeni R. More on Golytely (1982) Gastroenterology 83: 729-730

43. Battolla R, Catterina A, Cavalleri MG et al (1996) Il clisma monocontrasto previo lavaggio del colon nel paziente anziano. Radiol Med 91: 610-615

44. Cittadini G, Sardanelli F, De Cicco E et al (1998) Intestinal preparation to double-contrast barium enema: a new combination of sennosides with a colonic lavage solution (SELG®). Clin Radiol (in press)

45. Lazzaroni M, Petrillo M, Desideri S, Bianchi Porro G. (1993) Efficacy and tolerability of polyethylene glycol - electrolyte lavage solution with and without simethicone in the preparation of patients with inflammatory bowel disease for colonoscopy. Aliment Pharmacol Ther 7: 655-659

9   Is the cleansing enema a necessary ritual?

"Cleansing enemas are unglamorous and almost surely the most misunderstood and improperly performed procedure in clinical medicine". These words by Miller [1] point out quite rightly how little attention was paid in the past to the scientific and pragmatic rationale on which this so frequent and important clinical act is based. In fact, when given by inexperienced personnel, five enemas are required on average for a thorough cleansing of the colon [2].

Fundamentally, the cleansing enema aims at provoking the expulsion of fecal material in the colon by triggering a series of mass movements induced by the stimulation of colonic pressoreceptors through a mechanical distention. Therefore, theoretically, plain tap water could be enough for this purpose. In practice, however, this is more or less partially successful, depending on whether the whole set of conditions indicated herebelow are actually met, namely:

- an adequate amount of water is introduced;
- the introduction method is technically correct;
- the stimulation of pressoreceptors extends also and above all to the right colon and not only to the distal portion of the left colon, which is normally more sensitive to this stimulus.

Generally speaking, approximately minimum 2 liters of liquid are necessary in the adult. A temperature equal to body temperature is recommended. The pressure of the liquid column should not exceed the pressure normally present in a standard enema irrigator placed 50 cm above the bed where the patient is lying, and then progressively lifted up to 1 m. Otherwise spasm may develop, thus preventing the column from reaching the right colon.

If, despite this position, the patient still complains of pain due to the onset of spasm, the best thing to do is not to withhold the flow of liquid (which would worsen the situation), but to perform a siphoning maneuver, by lowering the tank below the decubitus plane. As soon as the spasm is over, the tank will be progressively raised again.

The patient, who starts in a prone decubitus, will progressively raise his/her right side until, midway during the enema, will have acquired a perfect left profile. Then, with a rapid movement, the patient will lie supine and will then slowly raise the left side until completion of the introduction of the liquid, at which stage he/she will be in perfect right profile. At this point the anal tip is removed and the patient is invited to turn himself/herself around once or twice and then to defecate.

This emergency situation which the colon has to face all of a sudden, triggers off two major defence mechanisms: 1. a whole series of mass movements through which the left colon is rapidly released of the just introduced contents, something which the right colon does much less frequently and in a more incomplete way; 2. an increase in normal liquid absorption, something in which the colon has limited capabilities (see Chapter 6).

Direct radiological experience has shown that the cleansing enema must be performed at least 45 minutes before the DCBE examination [3]. However, in practice, when the DCBE is performed less than 2-3 hours from the cleansing enema, in half of the patients a more or less significant dilution of the barium suspension is observed, the mucosa fails to be perfectly coated, while the presence of excessive barium/air levels is observed. This is mainly the case in the right colon, whereas the left colon seems not to be affected, probably due to the more effective peristaltic rushes induced in this part. The ultrasound examination of the cecum may offer a rapid and accurate method for detection of colonic water retention [4].

Colon inability to reabsorb residue liquids exceeding 1,400 mL in volume has also been demonstrated by the overall unsatisfactory experiences made with intestinal irrigation after gastric intubation and perfusion of about 6 liters of isotonic solution in 2 hours: abundant residues of liquid in the right colon; insufficient mucosal coating; significant alterations in the biochemical profile [5]. Better, yet still insufficient results for DCBE requirements are often obtained with a balanced electrolyte solution containing polyethylene glycol, Golytely, 4 liters of which are administered orally in the afternoon before the examination (see Chapter 8).

A possible way out could be the addition of some suitable components to the enema (i.e. bisacodyl, cascara sagrada, tannic acid) in order to induce a more complete and rapid evacuation. In our experience, intestinal cramping up to pain threshold and even lipothymia are a rather frequent consequence to the addition of contact laxatives. It is therefore advisable to use them only in the last cleansing enema performed the same morning of the X-ray examination under direct control of the radiologist. Furthermore, the induction of colon reactions, like those found in bowel motor neurosis, can be radiologically demonstrated. All in all, the improvement in evacuation results is not so significant to justify this procedure which makes the whole preparation more complex.

Much more satisfactory results can be obtained with tannic acid [6]. However, as already explained in Chapter 2, this substance was banned in 1964. Then, in 1972, at the strong request of radiologists, it was introduced again, but with certain restrictions on the admissible amount. The addition of 2.5 g of tannic acid to the cleansing enema is particularly beneficial since it allows the complete voiding of the cleansing fluid through the tonic contraction of the whole colon, and also for its astringent action on colonic mucosa which enhances barium suspension adhesion [7]. When the cleansing enema is judged to be essential, as is the case in elderly patients where the effect of purely pharmacological treatment is often insufficient [8, 9] it should be added with tannic acid, under direct control of the radiologist.

Whether cleansing enemas can lead to alterations of the sodium pump is still controversial. According to Plum and Dunning [10], every liter of introduced enema liquid, 7 mEq of K^+ are lost, specially when such a liquid is withheld longer than recommended above. However, this fact was not confirmed in the literature [11], nor by our personal data reported below. The effect is likely to depend on the amount of residual water after evacuation. Water carries Na^+ ions inside the cells: when the sodium pump is working properly, for every Na^+ ion entering the cell, a K^+ ion is expelled; a more or less significant intracellular K^+ loss ensues with concurrent excretion of HCO_3^- ions. These undesirable effects can be minimized by enriching the enema fluid with K^+ and HCO_3^-; conversely, the addition of NaCl mainly done to make the enema more isotonic, will yield the opposite effect.

In a research we have conducted to identify enema induced alterations in the biochemical profile [12], 18 healthy male volunteers, aged 24 to 56, have been investigated. After venous blood sampling, in the morning two hours after a light breakfast, a 2 liter tap water enema was performed. After 1, 3 (before lunch) and 24 hours from the enema, other venous blood samples were taken. Calcium, phosphorus, potassium and sodium ions, lactic-dehydrogenase, pyruvic transaminase, alkaline phosphatase, bilirubin, triglycerides, glucose, nitrogen, creatinine, uric acid, albumin and total proteins were evaluated. Important changes were observed for creatinine, triglycerides and lactic-dehydrogenase. A significant drop in creatinine serum values was observed in the first hour with almost a total recovery in the third hour (Fig. 1). A 15% drop in serum triglycerides was observed in the third hour, with a later return to normal basic values (Fig. 2). Conversely, lactic-dehydrogenase showed a sudden significant fall in the third and twenty-fourth hour (Fig. 3). It should be stressed that the cleansing enema has not significantly changed the chemical profile of the blood in treated individuals, at least with regard to the ions involved in the Na/K pump. No data are available on the effects of other enemas made within a short period of time, as generally done during preparation to the DCBE, for which up to 3-4 enemas are considered feasible [13].

Yet, it is not so much the concern about possible alterations in the blood biochemical profile, but rather several other considerations of different nature, which are urging a revision in the indiscrimi-

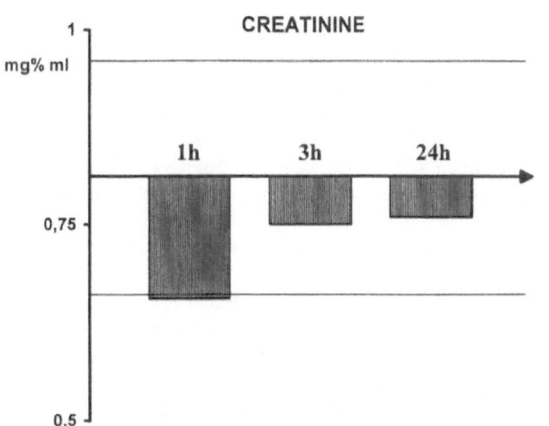

Fig. 1. Blood creatinine levels after cleansing enema in 18 male volunteers. The central line indicates the average basal level; the band above and below it represents the confidence interval (P = 0.05). Histograms show changes at 1, 3 and 24 hours, respectively, after the cleansing enemas

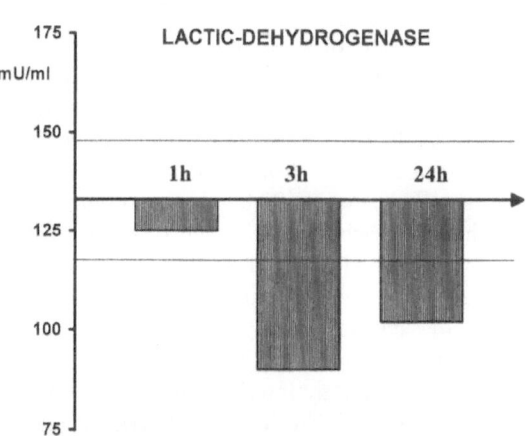

Fig. 3. Blood lactic-dehydrogenase levels after cleansing enema. See legend to Fig. 1

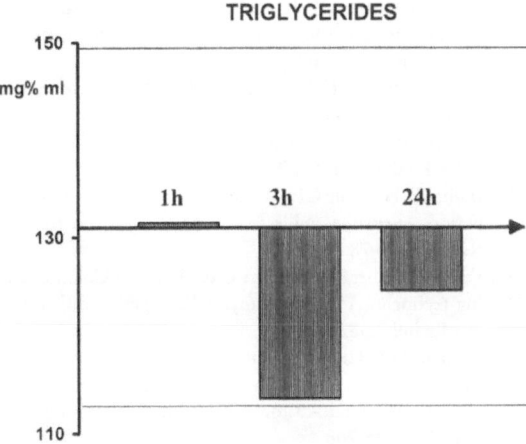

Fig. 2. Blood triglyceride levels and cleansing enema. See legend to Fig. 1

nate use of cleansing enemas. As more specifically discussed in Chapter 22, the cleansing enema is considered by the patient as a regressive submission act evoking a kind of mother/child interaction. An act to which he/she is not so prepared to submit as for the barium enema which he/she recognizes as a real diagnostic need. A long discussion on the need for such a cleansing enema may often take place, ending up with the patient submission to the will

of the physician, something which is internalized in an often unpredictable way.

When the patient is required to perform the enema himself/herself, it is often done improperly, also for the above mentioned reasons, and he/she will rarely admit it. Hence, the need to have it performed by paramedics to be suitably instructed also on the psychological aspects of such a treatment. In this case, paramedical staff will be overloaded with work, especially, paradoxically enough, in those centers where, for the high number of diagnostic examinations on the colon, their collaboration would be preferred in other tasks.

Therefore, a logic question would be: "Is the cleansing enema really necessary?". Historically, a long time has past since the first discussions on this topic, and, to say it with T.S. Eliot, there has been "time yet for a hundred indecisions, and for a hundred visions and revisions, before the taking of a toast and tea". But there is controversy yet as to the value of preparatory enema. Some regard it as useless [14-17], others suggest that it confers no benefit on the quality of the preparation [18,19], others consider it to be important [20,21]. Gelfand, Chen and Ott [22,23] define it crucial, and observe that it serves a threefold purpose: 1. it removes any remaining fecal material from the colon; 2. it allows to determine whether the colon is sufficiently clean to proceed with the examination (if not, the cleansing enema is repeated once or twice); 3. it indicates whether the patient can easily retain an enema (helping in part to determine whether a single- or double-contrast examination should be performed).

From a statistical point of view, according to the 1987 survey by Thoeni and Margulis [24], preparatory enemas are given slightly less frequently (42%) than in 1976 (56%). This percentage is likely to have gone down even further in the last years. In Italy, out of 400,000 barium examinations of the colon each year, a preparatory enema is done in no more than 10%. Therefore, our personal experience can be summarized in few words: no cleansing enema is necessary when the Genoa preparation protocol to DCBE is applied, since it may even negatively interfere on mucosal coating, probably through the removal of residual magnesium ions in the colon after the ingestion of the saline purgative.

However, no matter which is the individual attitude to the need of a cleansing enema: if actually performed, it has to be under the direct responsibility of a radiologist, since its execution may have too drastic positive or negative effects on DCBE resolution power.

References

1. Miller RE (1975) The cleansing enema. Radiology 117:483-485
2. Barnes MR (1969) Clean colons without enemas. Am J Nurs 69:2128
3. Lee SH, Bartram CI (1990) Determining the minimal interval between cleansing water enema and double-contrast barium enema examination. Clin Radiol 41:331-332
4. Pietila JA, Bondestam S, Hartel GJ et al (1990) The assessment of colonic water retention prior to double-contrast enema. Gastrointest Radiol 15:164-168
5. Bakran A, Bradley JA, Breshnihan E (1977) Whole gut irrigation: An inadequate preparation for double contrast barium enema examination. Gastroenterology 73:28-30
6. Welin S, Welin G (1976) The double contrast examination of the colon. Experience with the Welin modification. Stuttgart: Thieme
7. Murray L, Janower MD (1965) Tannic acid and the barium enema. Radiology 85:887
8. Tinetti ME, Stone L, Cooney L et al (1989) Inadequate barium enemas in hospitalized elderly patients. Incidence and risk factors. Arch Intern Med 149:2014-2016
9. Gurwitz JH, Noonan JP, Sanchez M et al (1992) Barium enemas in the frail elderly. Am J Med 92:41-44
10. Plum F, Dunning MF (1957) Enema-induced potassium loss in patients with disease of the spinal cord and cauda equina. Am J Med Sci 233:387-391
11. Welin S, Welin G, Aberg T (1970) Klyxray: a new preparation for excessive emptying of the colon. Br J Radiol 43:744-746
12. Oliva L, Cittadini G (1981) Il clisma a doppio contrasto: problemi metodologici e tecnici. Verona: Cortina
13. Pietila JA, Kinnunen J, Linden H (1990) The cleansing enema: How many for a good quality double-contrast enema? Acta Radiol 31:489-492
14. Rosengren JE, Aberg T (1975) Cleansing of the colon without enemas. Radiology 15:421-426
15. De Lacey G, Benson M, Wilkins R et al (1982) Routine colonic lavage is unnecessary for double-contrast barium enema in outpatients. BMJ 284:1021-1022
16. Hageman MJHH, Goei R (1993) Cleansing enema prior to double-contrast barium enema examination: is it necessary? Radiology 187:109-112
17. Chakraverty S, Hughes T, Keir MJ et al (1994) Preparation of the colon for double-contrast barium enema: Comparison of Picolax, Picolax with cleansing enema and Citramag (2 sachets) - A randomized prospective trial. Clin Radiol 49:566-569
18. Lee JR, Ferrando JR (1984) Variables in the preparation of the large intestine for double contrast barium enema examination. Gut 25:69-72
19. Mahieu PHG (1989) Compared evaluation of a new cleansing method of the colon before double contrast barium enema: Routine colonic lavage is no longer required. J Belge Radiol 72:475-479
20. Irwin JP, Peterson GH (1982) Colon preparation for the barium enema: A guide for the radiologist. Gastrointest Radiol 7:75-78
21. Fork FT, Ekberg G, Nilsson G et al (1982) Colon cleansing regimens: A clinical study in 1200 patients. Gastrointest Radiol 7:383-389
22. Gelfand DW, Chen YM, Ott DJ (1988) Colonic cleansing for radiographic detection of neoplasia: Efficacy of the magnesium citrate-castor oil-cleansing enema regimen. AJR 151:705-708
23. Gelfand DW, Chen YM, Ott DJ (1991) Preparing the colon for the barium enema examination. Radiology 178:609-613
24. Thoeni RF, Margulis AR (1988) The state of radiographic technique in the examination of the colon: A survey in 1987. Radiology 167:7-12

10 A simple, innocuous and effective method for cleansing the large bowel without enemas

A rational approach to the issue of bowel preparation for DCBE should induce to pursue several endpoints:

- radical cleansing of the colon with thorough removal of fecal matter without cleansing enemas;
- no major distress for the patient: this is a very important point when the aim is to allow the patient to carry out his/her normal activities until the DCBE examination;
- normal calorie diet: very important, especially in patients who have to undergo several diagnostic examinations within a short period of time;
- simple and accurate instructions comprehensible to the patient;
- simplification of the work of physicians and paramedics in charge of the examination.

In order to achieve the above objectives through pharmacological treatment alone, our group considered the following sequential actions [1]:

1. *administration of a first cathartic acting on the colon alone*: its effect should induce a defecation as much as possible similar to a spontaneous one (solid or maximum semisolid discharge);
2. *subsequent administration of a second cathartic acting on the small intestine alone,* which rapidly removes all the contents there, acting exactly when the previous purgative is exerting its effects on the colon;
3. *hydration of the patient* in order to limit loss of water which is frequent after intense cathartic treatment.

The mechanisms and action characteristics of available cathartics were examined and some of them have been directly tested. Our attention was drawn to some active principles of senna extracts

having exclusive action on the colon: sennosides A and B which, as purified crystals, are available in the form of calcium salts.

Sennoside A is formed by the dextrorotatory dianthronic aglycon sennidine A and D-glucose; *sennoside B* by compensated dianthronic aglycon mesosennidine B and D-glucose. These two sennosides, which are inactive as glucosides, after oral administration are absorbed by the small intestine, and become active through hydrolysis of the glucosidic bond, and later are excreted by the colon. Therefore, at the level of the emunctory (i.e. the colon) the first effects are felt after about 6 hours, exactly as desired. Twofold effects are observed: 1. direct stimulation of myenteric plexuses whereby effective mass propulsion movements are triggered; 2. intestinal sodium absorption inhibition, with subsequent water flow toward the lumen of the colon through osmosis. For the effective colonic mass movements induced and, at the same time, their limited number, sennosides can be considered as the optimal agents for the set objectives.

The emptying of the small intestine from the chyme there contained, a potential contaminator of the colon, is easily obtained with saline cathartics which have a less intense effect than castor oil and with which a more accurate dosage is possible.

Magnesium sulfate is practically perfect for this purpose. When orally administered in hypertonic form (15% w/v) it draws a sufficient amount of fluids to the intestinal lumen so as to stimulate the pressoreceptors on the intestinal wall. The effect is rapid, with recurrent liquid discharges for 2-3 hours after ingestion.

Hydration can be easily obtained by inviting the

patient to drink, as soon as the effects of the saline purgative begin, 1.5-2 liters of liquids (water, non-carbonated beverages, tea, camomile tea) in 2-3 hours.

With the above regimen and, above all, by strictly complying with the recommended dosage and schedule, all the contents of the small intestine are pushed into the colon exactly when its maximum propulsion activity is going on. Hence, all intestinal contents are pushed *vis a tergo* in a natural way rather than being "enveloped" as is the case with the cleansing enema. In this way, a better cleansing of the right colon is also ensured, which is generally more difficult to clean and, in 10-36% of cases, cannot even be reached by colonoscopy [2].

On the basis of this rationale, clinical testing was started, in a first phase, on adult individuals of both sexes to whom DCBE had been prescribed for suspected non acute organic colon diseases. The dose of sennosides was assessed on a trial and error base, so as to be sufficient to produce, after the ingestion of the cathartic with the morning breakfast, 2-4 mass propulsion movements starting from the same afternoon and lasting maximum until evening. An aqueous 1.5% w/v solution of a mixture of sennosides A and B calcium salts in equal parts was used for this purpose. This solution was kept in dark glass bottles with pierceable caps to protect it from light and air. Every time, only the required amount was taken and then mixed with the morning coffee, milk or tea. In order to avoid any use of other drugs, a cleansing enema was performed on each patient, the next morning, two hours before the X-ray examination. The right dose we were looking for resulted to be 150 mg. Patients had no abnormal sensations. The first colon movements start at around 2:00 p.m. leading, in the majority of cases, to a first solid discharge followed by a semisolid one. A third discharge is generally produced at about 9:00 p.m. The next morning a fourth discharge is often produced.

In a second phase, magnesium sulfate was also administered between the third and fourth hour after lunch, in such a quantity so as 3-4 liquid discharges would be produced in about 3 hours, the last of them practically without any fecal contents. The dose we were looking for resulted to be 15 g dissolved in half a glass of water. Isotonia is achieved with 400-500 mL of endogenous fluids. The patient is to be kept properly hydrated by inviting him/her to drink 250 mL of liquids every

twenty minutes between 5 and 8 p.m. The following morning no further preparation of the patient was required before DCBE examination.

Finally, controlled clinical testing was conducted on inpatients randomly subdivided to fall each of them into one of the two preparation protocols illustrated in Table 1.

Table 1. Preparation protocols under comparative evaluation

Group A

2 and 1 day before the examination: low-residue diet
1 day before:

8 a.m.	150 mg of sennosides at breakfast
1 p.m.	normal calorie lunch depending on the diet
4.30 p.m.	15 g magnesium sulfate in half a glass of lukewarm water
5 to 9 p.m.	1 glass of water every 30 minutes
9 p.m.	if necessary: one cup of clear soup

The morning of the examination: fast

Group B

2 and 1 day before the examination: low-residue diet
1 day before:

8 a.m.	cleansing enema (2 L water plus 15 g NaCl and 5 g NaHCO$_3$)
1 p.m.	normal calorie lunch depending on the diet
4 p.m.	50 ml castor oil
5 to 9 p.m.	1 glass of water every 30 minutes
9 p.m.	if necessary: one cup of clear soup
10 p.m.	cleansing enema

The morning of the examination: fast; 3 hours before: cleansing enema

Upon examination, each patient was required to give his/her impression on the treatment received and to report all side effects, even the minor ones. At the same time, the various effects produced were carefully checked against the theoretical assumptions, and an *a priori* judgement was made on the expected level of cleansing.

DCBE was performed according to the Altaras technique [3]. One mg of atropine sulfate was administered by mouth half an hour before the examination. The barium suspension (Barotrast 65% w/v) was introduced under fluoroscopic control up to the cecum. The patient was asked to take the appropriate decubitus positions to allow the removal of free surplus barium suspension in the lumen which was drained through the rectal tip. Immediately before colon insufflation, 20 mg of Buscopan were administered intravenously. Finally, 6 standard radiographs were taken, as envisaged by the "colon status" technique.

The obtained radiographs were examined by two skilled radiologists who did not know the type of preparation employed. A judgement was made on the cleansing level of the colon according to the following scoring:

Excellent = no appreciable fecal material
Good = minimal 1-2 mm diameter fecal residues
Fair = moderate fecal residues (up to 5 mm diameter)
Poor = appreciable fecal residues making difficult but not hindering diagnostic judgment
Unacceptable = significant fecal residues requiring to repeat the examination.

This experimental protocol was carried out on 182 inpatients, 86 of them prepared with the A protocol (sennosides + magnesium sulfate), 96 with the B protocol (castor oil + cleansing enemas).

The difference in the distribution of patients belonging to the two experimental groups among the five scoring classes was highly significant (χ^2 = 21.421; P < .001). The patients prepared with sennosides and magnesium sulfate tend to fall in the two upper classes (79% vs. 56.2% of Group B). The number of examinations which need to be repeated goes down from 8.3% (in patients prepared with castor oil and cleansing enemas) to 4.6% in Group A.

Only 8 out of 86 patients in group A spontaneously complained of excessively drastic effects (2 gastrectomized patients who had an early effect with diarrheal discharge already in the morning; 2 patients with diarrheal discharges during the night; 4 patients with abdominal cramping which, however, did not reach the threshold of abdominal pain). Therefore, taken all together, only 9.3% of patients have actually reported some problems worth mentioning. In Group B, 28% of patients have reported problems similar to those complained by the previous group, though with a higher incidence of abdominal cramping. Practically all of them expressed dislike for the cleansing enemas.

Two findings concerning Group A are worth mentioning. In 60% of cases, at the plain X-ray film of the abdomen which was routinely performed at the beginning of the procedure, an abnormal distribution of meteorism in the colon was observed, which tends to concentrate in the transverse colon that, in some cases, resulted to be moderately distended. This fact has no impact on barium adhesion to the colonic mucosa, but could become a problem when this preparation is used for other types of X-ray examinations, urography for example.

With regard to mucosal coating, it should be noted that, since some consistent magnesium sulfate residues are still present in the colon when the barium suspension is introduced, an interaction with the latter takes normally place, as discussed in greater detail in Chapter 15.

Considering the good agreement of the results obtained with the theoretical assumptions, in 1979 we decided to adopt our intestinal preparation protocol on a routine basis. This has so radically simplified the tasks of nurses in the hospital wards that complaints are constantly voiced, whenever there is the need to use, in individual patients, cleansing enemas for bowel preparation.

The popularity of the Genoa protocol was undoubtedly favored by the following elements:
- nurses in individual wards have become convinced of the validity of the technique and, therefore, are applying it more scrupulously;
- use of a proprietary drug, Pursennid (Sandoz, Basel, Switzerland), of which 13 tablets of 12 mg each are to be ingested, with a total sennosides A and B content of 156 mg. Less consistent results were obtained, in our hands, with X-Prep (Gray Pharmaceutical, Norwalk, Conn.), a standardized senna extract containing 142 mg of sennosides A and B in one single bottle;
- preparation regimen also applied to outpatients.

In children, where, as known, the use of cathartics and cleansing enemas is undesirable in constipation and clinically suspected Hirschsprung's disease, the Genoa technique has been successfully employed [4]. Personally, we believe that in children from 6 to 12 years of age the risk of severe diarrhea can be minimized by halving the dose of sennosides and with a 0.2 g/kg dose of magnesium sulfate.

In the elderly, we use the standard intestinal preparation without any modification. Should any significant amount of fecal material be identified by the fluoroscopic examination, the patient is invited to defecate, thus using the barium enema as a cleansing proper enema. If residual contrast medium is still sufficient, Buscopan is injected and insufflation performed, otherwise the colon is refilled and drained again according to the usual technique.

Often, as observed by Cargill and Hately [5], "the routines for preparation of the large bowel prior to radiological examination have come to be accepted by time hallowed tradition, and in some cases they are tolerated as barely satisfactory, rather than by any claim to excellence". The Genoa technique, with its 15 years strong implementation and with more than 41,500 DCBE examinations carried out in our Hospital, is, in our opinion, a significant progress towards a simple, innocuous and effective intestinal cleansing without cleansing enemas. For the valid results obtained, it has become a reference technique in the preparation to DCBE and, interestingly enough, it has been used also for colonoscopy [6] and in the preparation to colon surgery [7].

The most recent quality control of the Genoa protocol was carried out in 1996 on 477 outpatients undergoing DCBE (275 females, 24-93 y., median age 61 y.; 202 males, 16-90 y., median age 65 y.). Age distribution as indicated in Fig. 1 shows a clear prevalence of elderly patients.

During a preliminary interview, each patient was given detailed explanations on how to make the preparation. The following elements were assessed at the moment of the examination: compliance, mild and heavy complaints, opinion on protocol acceptability. Finally, the level of intestinal cleansing, mucosal coating and diagnostic reliability of the examination were assessed.

Full compliance was achieved in 86.2% of cases. Minor deviations from prescription, unlikely to bias the results, were recorded in 7.7% of cases. In the remaining 6.1% of cases, compliance was insufficient (no sennosides were taken in 1 case, reduced dose in 5 cases; no magnesium sulfate was taken in 5 cases, reduced dose in 5 cases; fluid intake of less than 1 liter in 10 cases; 3 patients had a cleansing enema, while 3 took castor oil, magnesium citrate and vegetable black, respectively).

No side effects were reported in 64.4% of patients; 27.4% reported mild side effects. The remaining 8.2% reported heavy side effects. Overall, the following side effects were reported, either alone or in association with other complaints: nausea by 12% of patients (2.5% with heavy nausea), vomiting by 5.3% (2.1% with heavy vomiting), abdominal cramping by 27.6% (6.1% with heavy cramping), insomnia by 1.7% (0.6% with heavy insomnia).

Fifty-two point eight percent of patients said that they liked the Genoa protocol, 45.5% said that it was acceptable and 1.7% of them said that they would not repeat the procedure in the future.

By overall judgment, intestinal cleansing was considered to be valid (excellent, good, fair) in 86.1% of patients, poor (but with sufficient examination reliability) in 9.9%, and unacceptable (with indication to repeat the examination) in 4% of patients (Fig. 2).

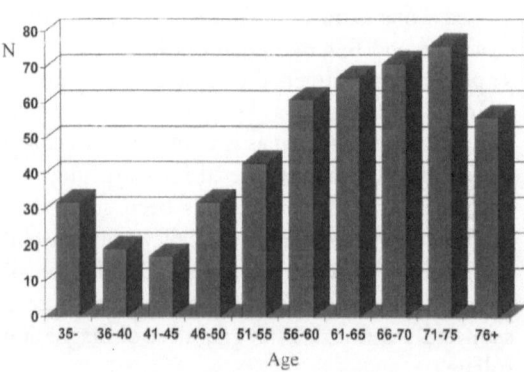

Fig. 1. Quality control of the Genoa protocol conducted in 1997. Age distribution of the 477 outpatients examined

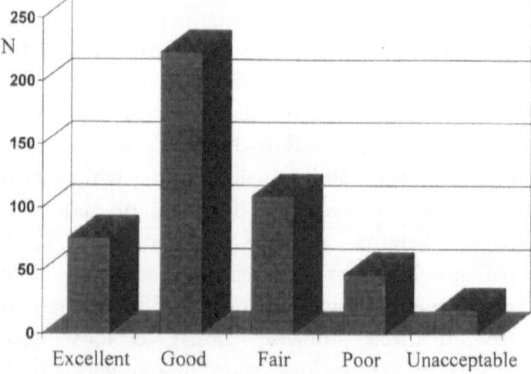

Fig. 2. Quality control of the Genoa protocol conducted in 1997. Colon cleansing levels obtained

Comparison tests were conducted between male and female patients and among the various age groups with Kruskal-Wallis one-criterion analysis of variance by ranks [8]. No difference (P = .50) was observed in cleansing level between males and females. Maximum cleansing, which decreases with age, was obtained in patients from 41 to 45 years old.

Cleansing levels in elderly patients overlap those of juvenile patients (Fig. 3). However, the observed differences are not statistically significant (P = .39).

Mucosal coating, which is a fundamental parameter for successful examination, resulted to be excellent or good in 93.9% of patients, and borderline or poor in 6.1%. No correlation was found with either patient gender or age.

Ninety-four point one percent of examinations were judged to be reliable for diagnostic purposes.

Several possible changes to the Genoa protocol have been tried in order to improve intestinal cleansing. Significant results have been obtained by associating sennosides with a proprietary iso-osmotic electrolyte solution containing polyethylene glycol (Selg, Promefarm, Milan, Italy - see Chapter 8). Some personal experimental data are worth a few considerations also because they allow a better comparison with the most popular endoscopic protocol for intestinal preparation [9].

Three hundred and sixty nine patients were randomly allocated to receive: 4 liters of Selg in the late afternoon, i.e. the usual endoscopic protocol, and 3 Dulcolax 5 mg tablets in the evening (group A); or 156 mg of sennosides at 8 a.m., 15 g of magnesium sulfate at 5 p.m., and subsequent hydration with 2 liters of water, i.e. the usual Genoa protocol (group B); or 156 mg of sennosides at 8 a.m. and 2 liters of Selg in the late afternoon (group C). DCBE examinations were performed with the Genoa technique employing Polybar ACB 57% w/v. Compliance of the protocol, complaints, cleansing (ranked as excellent, good, fair, poor, unacceptable), mucosal coating (ranked as excellent, good, thin diagnostic, borderline, insufficient), and amount of fluid retained in the colon lumen were independently evaluated by two radiologists. Kruskal-Wallis test on ranks and chi-square test were used to evaluate significance of the results.

Compliance was satisfactory in every group. A higher incidence of nausea was observed in group A, of abdominal cramping in group C. Colon cleansing was better in group C than both in group A (P = .0002) and in group B (P = .0220). Mucosal coating was better in group B than both in group A (P = .0049) and C (P < .0001). Air/barium levels were higher in group C than in group A (P = .0048) and B (P = .0053). Diagnostic accuracy was good in every group.

The combination of sennosides and Selg raises to an interesting level colonic cleansing vs. both the Genoa and the endoscopic protocol (Fig. 4). In particular, a perfect cleansing is achieved in 33.3% of cases, a good cleansing in 49% and a fairly good cleansing in 14.6% as against 23.5, 51 and 15.3%, respectively, of the Genoa protocol and 9.4, 68.8 and 15.6% of the endoscopic protocol. The examination has to be repeated only in 3.8% of cases.

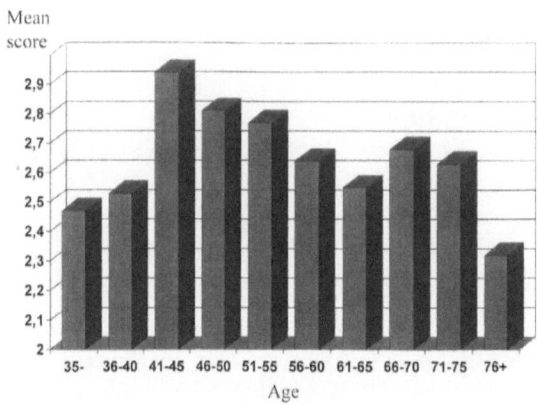

Fig. 3. Quality control of the Genoa protocol conducted in 1997. Mean scores for intestinal cleansing obtained in the various age groups

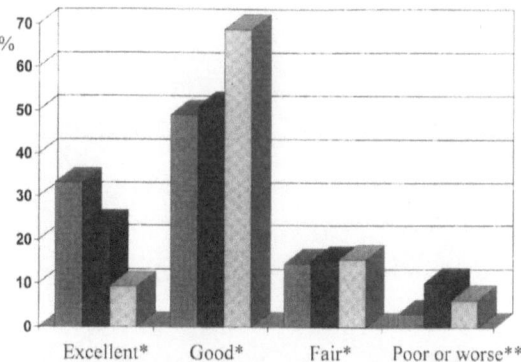

Fig. 4. Colonic cleansing levels obtained with sennosides and Selg (middle gray), sennosides and magnesium sulfate (dark gray), Selg and Dulcolax (light gray). *at least one observer; **both observers

Thus, 96.2% of the examinations have diagnostic value, versus 89.8% with the Genoa protocol and 93.7% with the endoscopic protocol.

The sennosides/Selg combination, which is still under experimental testing, is a variation from the Genoa protocol that is definitely asserting itself on the field. It is particularly safe and effective in elderly and debilitated patients, as well as in patients with cardiac, renal or pulmonary diseases.

References

1. Cittadini G, Rollandi GA, Giribaldi M (1980) Su un metodo semplice innocuo ed efficiente di pulizia intestinale senza clisteri. Radiol Med 66:415-420
2. Mac Carty RL (1992) Colorectal cancer: The case for barium enema. Mayo Clin Proc 67(3):253-257
3. Altaras J. (1982) Radiologischer Atlas, Kolon und Rektum. München: Urban & Schwarzenberg
4. Tamburrini O, Del Vecchio E, Sodano A (1983) Clisma in età pediatrica - Tecnica e metodica. Napoli: Idelson, pp 19-24
5. Cargill A, Hately W (1978) Preparation of the colon prior to radiology - a comparison of the effectiveness of castor oil, Dulcodos and X-Prep liquid. Br J Radiol 51:910-912
6. Pugliese V, Bruzzi P, Aste H (1982) Left-sided colonoscopy in screening programs: What preparation? Endoscopy 14:85-88
7. Cafiero F, Sertoli MR, Rubagotti A et al (1981) La preparazione antibiotica negli interventi sul grosso intestino: Studio sperimentale. Minerva Chir 36:941-943
8. Kruskal WH, Wallis WA (1952) Use of ranks in one-criterion variance analysis. J Am Statistic Assoc 47: 583-621
9. Cittadini G, Sardanelli F, De Cicco E et al (1998) Intestinal preparation to double-contrast barium enema: a new combination of sennosides with a colonic lavage solution (SELG®). Clin Radiol (in press)

11 Effects of antimuscarinic drugs on the colon

Tone, motility and secretion of the colon are under the control of the autonomic nervous system. Under the stimulation of the *parasympathetic system*, a marked increase in tone and motility is recorded, together with an increase in secretion and sphincter relaxation. Conversely, under the stimulation of the *sympathetic system*, tone and motility are slightly reduced, with secretion inhibition and sphincter contraction. Parasympathetic innervation becomes particularly important in DCBE, for the greater control it exerts on the above mentioned colon functions, which may significantly affect the results of the examination, and also because these effects can be easily inhibited with appropriate drugs.

The cecum, ascending and transverse colon are innervated by the parasympathetic fibers of the nervus vagus; the descending colon, sigmoid and rectum are innervated by the pelvic nerves. Acetylcholine (Fig. 1) is the neurotransmitter at the level of preganglionic synapses, where it interacts with *nicotinic cholinergic receptors* (consisting of at least two different pentameric proteins). Its action is electively blocked by ganglioplegics. Acetylcholine is also active at the synapses between postganglionic fibers and effector cells through *muscarinic cholinergic receptors* (consisting of at least five different glycoproteins having different anatomic sites and peculiar chemical features); its action is electively blocked by atropine and other antimuscarinic drugs. It is important to remember that the intrinsic electrical and mechanical activity of the colonic smooth muscles is modified, but not triggered, by neural input [1].

Antimuscarinic or atropinic drugs - also called spasmolytics for their inhibiting effect on the smooth muscles - when administered in therapeutic dose, essentially act as acetylcholine competitive antagonists at the muscarinic receptor level. They induce local-

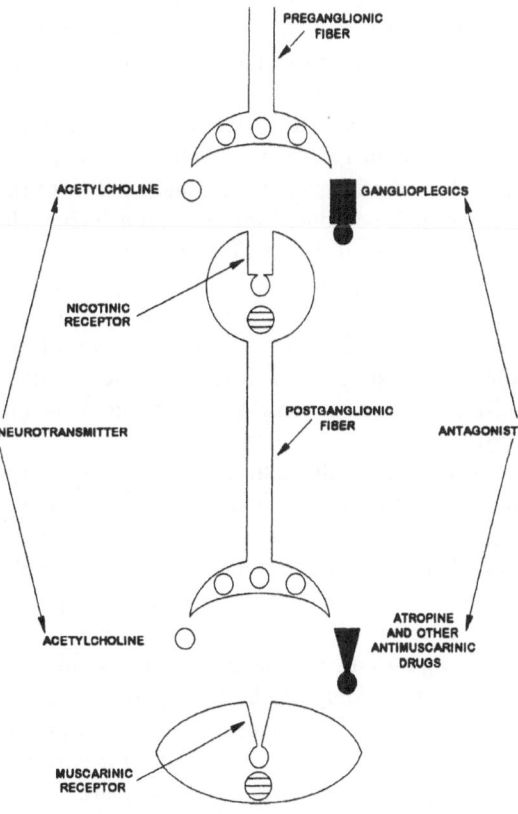

Fig. 1. Parasympathetic innervation of the colon. Neurotransmitters and impulse antagonists at the level of the synapse

ized effects on the effector cells in the various body districts (myocardium, smooth muscles, glands) innervated by postganglionic parasympathetic fibers. However, when administered in therapeutic doses, their antagonist action at the level of ganglionic nicotinic receptors is modest, and even lower on nicotinic receptors of the neuromuscular plate. Yet, the effect of antimuscarinic drugs containing quaternary ammonium compounds on nicotinic receptors is greater than those without such compounds.

In the central nervous system, cholinergic transmission is mainly nicotinic in the spinal cord and muscarinic at cortical and subcortical level. Therefore, the initially stimulating and then depressing effects of atropinic drugs on the central nervous system are felt at the level of the cortex and subcortical structures. Conversely, with quaternary ammonium compounds, which hardly cross the blood-brain barrier, these effects are lacking or minimal.

Not all effector cells innervated by the parasympathetic system are equally sensitive to antimuscarinic agents. Atropine, in small doses, has a depressing action on salivary, bronchial secretion and sweating; in greater doses, dilatation of the pupil, accommodation paralysis and tachycardia are induced (Table 1). Only with even greater doses, is the parasympathetic control on the digestive tract (with subsequent reduction in gastroenteric tone and motility) and on the bladder (with urination difficulty) lost. Gastric secretion can be inhibited only with even greater doses. Therefore, it is evident that, in principle, the tone and motility of the colon cannot be reduced without also reducing salivary and bronchial secretion and sweating, and without causing dilatation of the pupil, accommodation alterations, tachycardia and hampered bladder emptying. However, with the majority of antimuscarinic drugs used in clinical practice, these adverse reactions are only mild, asymptomatic and transient.

Genes which codify muscarinic cholinergic receptors with different structures and capable of inducing specific functional response have been demonstrated in humans [2], thus making it possible in the future to produce antimuscarinic drugs with greater organ selectivity than those currently available [1].

Though some antimuscarinic drugs, like atropine, are capable of eliminating the effects of acetylcholine and parasympathomimetic drugs on the gastrointestinal tract, they inhibit the effects of parasympathetic stimulation only partially. This is the case particularly in the colon, since other neurotransmitters, co-transmitters and neuromodulators (i.e. purines, eicosanoids, peptides) locally produced by enteric neurons, are involved [1].

Table 1. Dose related atropine effects

0.25 mg (i.m. or s.c. - max effect after 30'-50') slight dryness of the mouth (salivary secretion reduction) mild bradycardia sweating reduction
0.5-1 mg dryness of the mouth modest tachycardia (sometimes preceded by bradycardia) modest dilatation of the pupil reduction in gastroenteric tone and motility
1.5 mg marked dryness of the mouth marked tachycardia (sometimes preceded by bradycardia) marked dilatation of the pupil paralysis of accommodation reduction in gastroenteric tone, motility and secretion hampered bladder emptying (due to detrusor urinae paralysis)

With oral atropine administration, the effects take place later and are slightly less marked

Since the effects of the various antimuscarinic drugs differ only quantitatively, it is sufficient to examine those of atropine, a well proven drug for its widespread use as pre-anaesthetic, and of hyoscine N-butylbromide (Buscopan, Boehringer Ingelheim), a quaternary ammonium compound, which is very commonly used in clinical practice as antispasmodic agent on the intestinal tract (Fig. 2).

Atropine pharmacokinetics has recently been studied through accurate experimental investigations on humans [3], which explained many of its properties after oral or parenteral administration as well as observed age-dependent effects of its action and some unwanted effects in very young and very old patients [4-6].

In adults, absorption of orally administered atropine, mainly occurring in the duodenum and jejunum, is practically total. Before entering into general circulation, atropine is in part metabolized in the liver to inactive compounds. Its maximum plasma concentration is reached 1 h after oral ad-

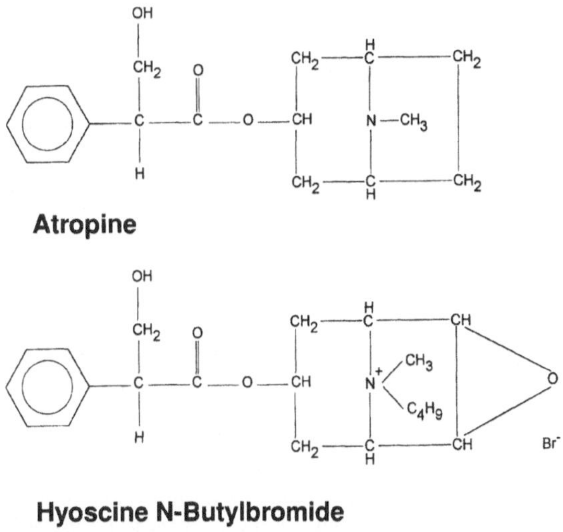

Atropine

Hyoscine N-Butylbromide

Fig. 2. Atropine and hyoscine N-butylbromide structure. It should be noted that the main difference between the two substances is not in the tropic acid component (*on the left*), but in the basic component (*on the right*), featuring tropine and scopine, respectively. Slightly ganglioplegic properties are attributed to the latter substance by the presence of quaternary nitrogen

ministration, and 15-50 minutes after i.m. administration with a 2.5 and 2 hours half-life, respectively. Typical peripheral antimuscarinic effects reach a peak after 2-4 hours and 1-2 hours, respectively. Generally speaking, the oral dose of atropine should be at least twice as high as the intramuscular one to produce the same peripheral effects. Ocular effects have a delayed onset with maximum after 6 hours. From 35 to 50% of atropine is excreted with the urine, the remaining is partly demethylated and partly conjugated with glycuronic acid.

In children under 2 and in the elderly, a high sensitivity to the effects of atropine, mainly those related to the central nervous system, may be observed. This seems to be linked to an increased distribution volume in children and a lowered clearance in the elderly [7]. Since in elderly people cardiovascular response to atropine is lower than in adults, alterations in the receptor sensitivity of different organs with increasing age must be invoked in addition to pharmacokinetic changes.

All in all, full therapeutic doses of atropine sulfate have clear and prolonged effects on colon motor activity, with reduction in tone, amplitude and frequency of peristaltic contractions. With a 0.8 mg i.m. dose, atropine inhibits, but could even to-

tally eliminate, colon tone and propulsion movements. However, in clinical practice, atropine is ever more rarely used as hypotonic drug in DCBE examination, since its action is not sufficiently targeted on the colon. Therefore, any valuable effect thus obtained for image improvement is limited by the extent of side effects. In addition, there are significant differences in individual response to the drug.

Similarly to atropine, *hyoscine N-butylbromide* is a competitive antagonist of acetylcholine at postganglionic parasympathetic nerve endings, where it exerts a blocking effect on muscarinic receptors. It has no effect on nicotinic receptors. Like all quaternary ammonium compounds, it does not cross the blood-brain barrier and hence, unlike atropine, it has no central effects. Peripheral anticholinergic effects are somewhat less pronounced and of shorter duration than with atropine. In humans, following administration of 20 mg i.v. there is a reduction in salivation, a transient increase in heart rate and a slight disturbance in visual accommodation lasting about 1 hour, with peak activity respectively 1.5%, 3% and 7.5% that of atropine [8].

The drug is partially metabolized in the liver to inactive compounds. Its excretion is more or less equal in the urine and in the feces. Intestinal absorption is low and only very small amounts are involved in entero-hepatic circulation.

A study on Buscopan effects on gut motility in humans [9] showed that with an 8 mg i.v. injection, peristalsis is reduced for about 15-30 minutes (in the first 6 minutes it is almost totally absent). In the following hour, an increased peristaltic activity follows the initial reduction, reaching its peak 50-60 minutes from the injection. Sometimes, a paradoxical increase in intestinal motility can take place immediately after injection. No effects on colon motility are observed with a 200 mg oral administration.

Owing to the rarity of severe adverse effects [10,11] and to the mild and transitory symptomatic adverse effects such as dryness of the mouth, tachycardia and visual blurring [12,13], Buscopan is very popular in clinical practice in Europe as an antispasmodic agent on the intestinal, biliary and urinary tract, and in spasmodic dysmenorrhea. It is also largely used as a hypotonic agent in radiological and endoscopic examination of the gastrointestinal tract [14,15], and prior to induction of anesthesia.

With regard to ocular effects induced by Buscopan, small measurable effects on near vision are observed in 13.5% of patients, but the degree of visual impairment is not sufficient to affect driving ability [16]. In general, a history of glaucoma is a contraindication to the use of Buscopan with the aim to avoid the rare development of acute closed-angle glaucoma. However, withholding Buscopan from these patients may unnecessarily restrict diagnostic capability [17]. The patient should rather be advised of the very low risk of developing acute glaucoma and warned to seek early medical advice if he/she should experience sudden eye pain or loss of vision in the first few hours following administration of Buscopan.

The efficacy of *hyoscine N-cyclopropylmethyl bromide* has been reported as a hypotonic drug inducing increased colonic distention and decreased motility, thus significantly improving image quality in DCBE [18]. More recently, similar results have been reported for *pirenzepine* [19]. However, these atropine-like antimuscarinic drugs are not yet popular in radiology.

References

1. Goodman LS, Gilman A. (1990) The pharmacological basis of therapeutics. 8th edition. New York: Pergamon Press
2. Bonner TI, Buckley NJ, Young AC et al (1987) Identification of a family of muscarinic acetylcholine receptors genes. Science 237:527-532
3. Kanto J, Klotz U (1988) Pharmacokinetic implications for the clinical use of atropine, scopolamine and glycopyrrolate. Acta Anaesthesiol Scand 32:69-78
4. Shutt LE, Bowes JB (1979) Atropine and hyoscine. Anaesthesia 134:476-479
5. Berg JM, Brandon MW, Kirman BH (1959) Atropine in mongolism. Lancet 2:441
6. Smith DS, Orkin FK, Gardner SM et al (1979) Prolonged sedation in the elderly after intraoperative atropine administration. Anesthesiology 51:348-349
7. Virtanen R, Kanto J, Iisalo E et al (1982) Pharmacokinetic studies on atropine with special refernce to age. Acta Anaesthesiol Scand 26:297-300
8. Herxheimer A, Haefeli L (1966) Human pharmacology of hyoscine butylbromide. Lancet 2:418-421
9. Guignard JP, Herxheimer A, Greenwood RM (1968) Effects of hyoscine butylbromide on gut motility. Clin Pharmacol Ther 9:745-748
10. Thomas AMK, Kubie AM, Britt RP (1986) Acute angioneurotic oedema following a barium meal. Br J Radiol 59:1055-1056
11. Treweeke P, Barrett NK (1987) Allergic reaction to Buscopan (letter). Br J Radiol 60:417-418
12. Herxheimer A, De Groot AC (1977) Some effects of injected hyoscine butylbromide: a versatile class experiment in human pharmacology. Br J Clin Pharmacol 4:337-342
13. Hüpscher DN, Dommerholt O (1984) Action and side effects of small doses of Buscopan in gastroduodenal radiography. Diagn Imaging Clin Med 53:77-86
14. Kreel L (1975) Pharmaco-radiology in barium examinations with special reference to glucagon. Br J Radiol 48:691-703
15. Lee JR (1982) Routine use of hyoscine N-butylbromide (Buscopan) in double contrast barium enema examinations. Clin Radiol 33:273-276
16. Sissons GRJ, McQueenie A, Mantle M (1991) The ocular effects of hyoscine-n-butylbromide ("Buscopan") in radiological practice. Br J Radiol 64:584-586
17. Doran RML, Gray R, Virjee JP (1987) Buscopan and glaucoma (letter). Br J Radiol 60:417
18. Golfieri G, Porta E, Imbimbo BP et al (1988) Efficacy of cimetropium bromide as pre-medication for double-contrast barium enema. Br J Radiol 61:1087-1088
19. Marraccini P, Braccini G, Marrucci A et al (1996) Pirenzepine versus scopolamine methyl bromide in double-contrast barium enema study of the large bowel. Abdom Imaging 21:304-308

12 Colonic pressure values after administration of atropine, buscopan and glucagon

Induction of colon hypotony is an important act for the radiologist before a DCBE examination. Through the reduction of colon segmentation thus obtained, the backward progress of the barium suspension inside the intestinal lumen is promoted, the large bowel is better distended during air insufflation, hence quality of the double-contrast images is improved.

In the Genoa technique, colon hypotony is induced by partially following the approach first proposed by Welin [1] and confirmed by several other Authors: i.e. drugs like atropine sulfate and Buscopan are administered which specifically inhibit the parasympathetic component of the autonomic nervous system by blocking its muscarinic receptors. Atropine is administered orally 40 minutes prior to the beginning of the examination, only when prevention of vagal reflexes and reduction in colonic mucosal secretion are recommended. Buscopan is administered intravenously in all patients immediately prior to gaseous distention of the colon. See Chapter 11 for detailed description of types of actions and pharmacokinetics of these two drugs.

The parameters adopted by radiologists to assess colon hypotony have often proved inaccurate and insufficient. Variations in colon tone cannot be properly assessed through fluoroscopy during barium enema examination, first of all because such assessment depends on the skills and observation capability of the radiologist performing the examination, and also because the motorial behavior of the large bowel under normal conditions is entirely different from the one observed under distention and stimulation by a foreign fluid. Hence, no standard interpretation is possible which would objectively guarantee the validity of detected parameters.

Based on this assumption, by using colonic manometry we decided to examine the behavior of colon intraluminal pressure in normal subjects in natural conditions as well as after atropine and Buscopan administration. In this way, the extent of wall tone variations induced by these drugs can objectively be assessed in the distal tract of the large bowel.

Intraluminal pressure values have been measured with an open-tip recording probe of original design, 60 cm length and 10 mm external diameter. The probe, after proper positioning inside the colon, is connected, by means of transducers, to a polygraph for the simultaneous plotting of motor behavior of the descending colon, sigmoid, rectum and anal sphincters.

In a first group of normal individuals (12 females and 8 males, mean age 38 years), the pressure values were plotted in basal conditions and, after i.m. administration of 1 mg atropine sulfate (12 patients) or i.v. administration of 20 mg Buscopan (8 patients), their evolution was followed for one hour (Figs. 1, 2). In a second group of normal individuals (3 females and 4 males, mean age 36 years) the combined action of both drugs was assessed following the same procedure. After plotting their basal pressure values, atropine was administered according to the same procedure described above, and after 30 minutes of plotting Buscopan was given. The interval in the administration of the two drugs was calculated so as to get the exact time of greatest atropine-induced hypotony, to see whether Buscopan would be able to further enhance the colon muscles relaxation previously induced by at-

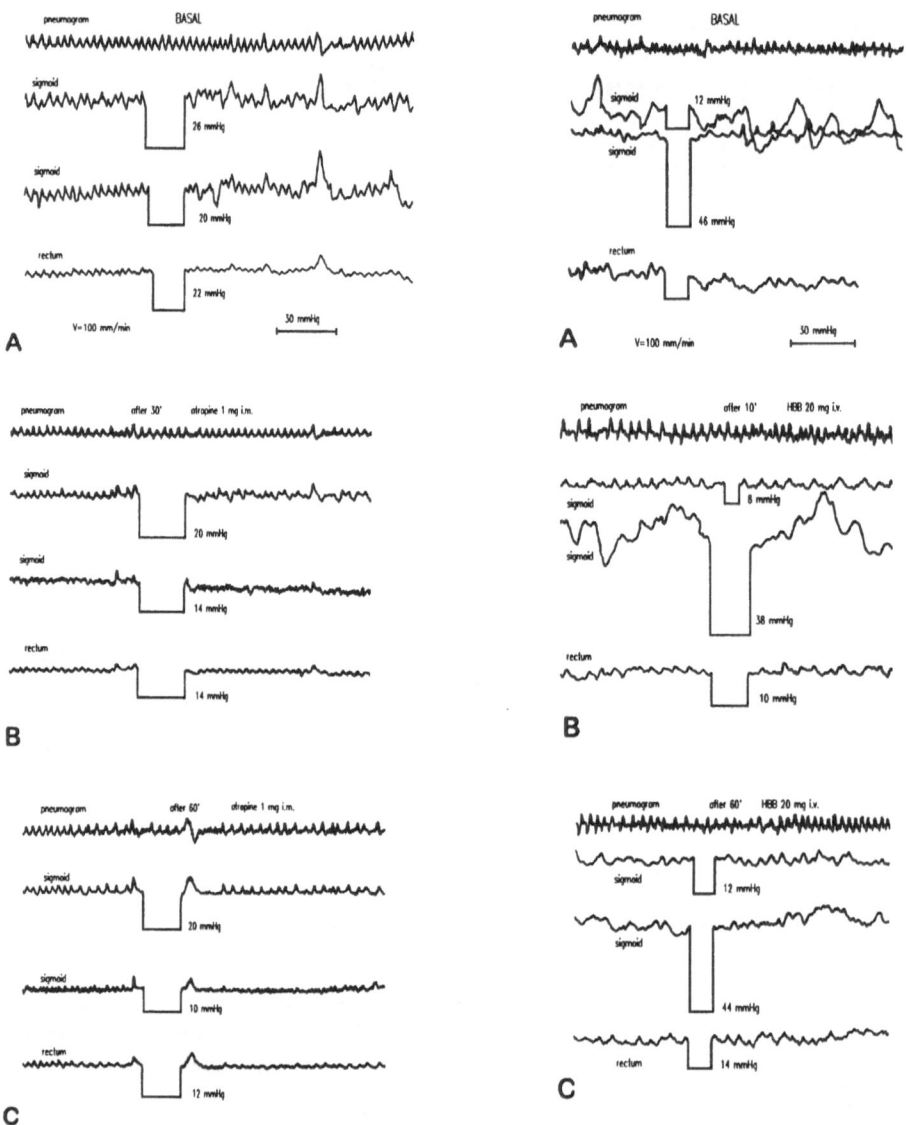

Fig. 1. Intraluminal pressure plotting in the rectum and sigmoid colon in basal conditions **(A)** and 30 **(B)** and 60 **(C)** minutes after i.m. administration of 1 mg atropine sulfate

Fig. 2. Intraluminal pressure plotting in the rectum and sigmoid colon in basal conditions **(A)** and 10 **(B)** and 60 **(C)** minutes after i.v. administration of 20 mg Buscopan

Table 1. Extracolic effects after i.m. 1 mg atropine administration

	10'	20'	30'	40'	50'	60'
Pupil reflex		−	− −	− −	− −	− −
Heart rate	−	+	+	++	+	+
Blood pressure				+	+	
Mouth dryness		+	++	++	++	++

+ Increase   - Decrease

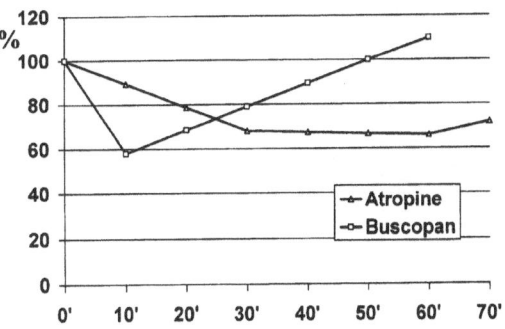

Fig. 3. Average percentage variations in intraluminal pressure values of the rectum-sigmoid after administration of atropine sulfate (1 mg i.m.) or Buscopan (20 mg i.v.)

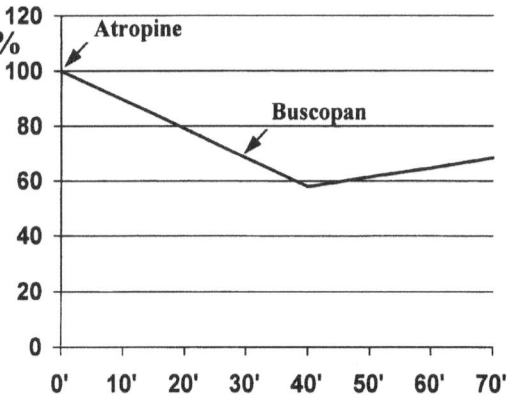

Fig. 4. Average percentage variations in intraluminal pressure values of the rectum-sigmoid after combined sequential administration (30 minutes interval) of atropine sulfate (1 mg i.m.) and Buscopan (20 mg i.v.)

ropine. The percentage variations from basal values in average intraluminal pressure values in three different points of the large bowel under examination are reported in Figs. 3 and 4. During the pressure analysis, pupil reflex, heart rate, arterial blood pressure, mouth dryness have also been assessed in each of the subjects in both groups (Table 1).

Atropine and Buscopan, when administered alone, have reduced the intraluminal pressure values by 34% and 42%, respectively (Fig. 3). With regard to atropine, its already significant effect after 30 minutes reaches its peak after 50-60 minutes, and then progressively dwindles in the following 60 minutes. Buscopan effect, which is more rapid, reaches its peak after 10 minutes, and wears out progressively during the following 30-40 minutes.

In the combined sequential administration of both drugs, Buscopan has reduced colon intraluminal pressure (already abated by atropine) by about

8% (Fig. 4). Therefore, though the total hypotonic effect is practically the same as with Buscopan alone, its kinetics is totally different.

The explanation for the limited hypotonic effect on the large bowel of antimuscarinic drugs is still complex and conjectural. For sure it can be said that tone and motility of the large bowel are under the control of the sympathetic-parasympathetic system for no more than 40%, and that an important role is played by complex intramural and peripheral nervous interaction mechanisms [2].

Preganglionic vagal fibers have synapses with cholinergic postganglionic fibers as well as with a network of intramural noncholinergic neurons making up the enteric plexus. Chemical mediators other than acetylcholine and capable of transmitting, *in vivo*, impulses exciting colon tone and motility are active on these intramural neurons [3].

Furthermore, smooth muscle fibercells are hyperpolarized by purinergic intramural neurons under the action of the parasympathetic system, thus leading to a paradoxical wall muscle relaxation [4]. The inferior mesenteric ganglion can also affect large bowel motility through a complex integration action of central neural inputs reaching it through splanchnic nerves and peripheral nervous inputs, reaching it through afferent fibers from lumbar spine segments and pelvic nervous ganglia [5].

It is worth mentioning that manometric assessments conducted with the same approach described above on normal subjects (4 females and 3 males, average age 35 years) before and after i.v. administration of 1 or 2 mg of glucagon failed to identify any variations in intraluminal pressure values. The hypotonic effect of this drug will be specifically discussed in Chapter 13.

References

1. Welin S (1958) Modern trends in diagnostic roentgenology of the colon. Br J Radiol 31:453-464
2. Wood JD (1975) Neurophysiology of Auberbach's plexus and control of intestinal motility. Physiol Rev 55:170-174
3. Szurszewski JH, Weems WA (1976) A study of peripheral input to and its control by post-ganglionic neurones of the inferior mesenteric ganglion. J Physiol 256:541-556
4. Gonella J (1978) La motilité digestive et sa regulation nerveuse. J Physiol 74:131-138
5. Weems WA, Szurszewski JH (1977) Modulation of colonic motility by peripheral neural inputs to neuron of the inferior mesenteric ganglion. Gastroenterology 73:273-289

13 Glucagon and the colon

Francesco Sardanelli

The use of glucagon in gastrointestinal radiology began in 1968 as hypotonic agent in duodenography [1] and was soon extended to the treatment of acute diverticulitis [2], as adjuvant in the endoscopic retrieval of biliary calculi [3], in esophageal food impaction [4,5], in the reduction of ileocolic intussusception [6-10], in the differential diagnosis between obstructive and hepatocellular jaundice [11], and above all in the radiographic examination of the gastrointestinal tract [12-14].

With regard to the radiographic examination of the colon, according to the survey by Thoeni and Margulis [14], the use of glucagon in the United States, where it is commonly employed in 82.7% of institutions, increased 20% between 1976 and 1987. Glucagon is administered selectively to distinguish between spasm and stenosis; it decreases discomfort during the examination, helps to retain the barium and it is useful for spastic colon. Glucagon is much less popular in Europe, where Buscopan is the most commonly used hypotonic drug. Is this only due to a free choice between two similar drugs, or is it due to different rationales for colon management during double-contrast barium enema examination?

Glucagon is a straight-chain polypeptide hormone containing 29 amino acid residues with a molecular weight of 3483. It is synthesized from a precursor, preproglucagon, which undergoes a sequential tissue-specific maturation with production of different glucagon-like secretory peptides in pancreas α-cells and in α-like intestinal cells [15]. Glucagon secretion, controlled by the autonomic nervous system, is increased by the stimulation from sympathetic nerves, and by the administration of sympathetic agonists and acetylcholine.

Glucagon stimulates hyperglycemia by promoting the breakdown of liver glycogen and the release of glucose into the circulation. It induces lipolysis, positive inotropic action on the heart, intestinal tone and motility reduction. Its effects are due to the interaction at the surface of the target cell with adrenergic receptors and are mediated, perhaps with the exception of the intestine, by activation of adenylate cyclase with consequent production of cyclic AMP. Glucagon is metabolized in the liver, kidneys, plasma and action sites; its half-life in the plasma is 3-6 minutes [16].

Commercially available glucagon is extracted from bovine or porcine pancreas, or genetically engineered through recombinant DNA technology.

Glucagon is usually administered by intravenous injection. At 0.25 to 2 mg, within one minute it produces its effect lasting for 9 to 25 minutes. Nausea and vomiting may occur in 10-15% of patients. It should be administered with caution to patients with insulinoma or pheochromocytoma as it induces hypoglycemia - due to its insulin-releasing effect [17,18] – and marked hypertension – due to subsequent catecholamine release [19] –, respectively. Caution is also required when it is employed as diagnostic aid in diabetic patients.

The polypeptide constituting glucagon is not thought to be allergenic, but may be contaminated by proteins providing the potential for allergic reactions [20, 21]. Consequently, repeated injections must be considered with particular attention. In fact, product information supplied by the manufacturer warns that generalized allergic reactions, including urticaria, respiratory distress, and hypotension, have been reported in patients who have received glucagon injection [22].

Following administration of exogenous glucagon, exocrine effects may appear, such as marked reduction in pancreatic juice secretion [23], inhibition of gastric acid secretion [24], of gastric and intestinal motility [25], stimulation of the flow of bile [26], of Brunner's glands and intestinal secretion [27]. In clinical practice, glucagon is used in the treatment of severe hypoglycemia in diabetics, shock, and for various painful gastrointestinal disorders associated with spasm.

Few doubts seem to exist about the satisfactory degree of hypotony and hypomotility induced on the stomach [12], duodenum [1, 12, 28-32], and small intestine [29, 30] by 0.25-0.5 mg glucagon given intravenously (with the following decreasing sensitivity order: duodenum, jejunum, stomach), and on the relaxation of the lower esophageal sphincter [33] and ileocecal valve [34-36] induced by 1-2 mg glucagon. Conversely, there is less agreement on glucagon effects on the large bowel [37] (apparently less responsive than the stomach [38]).

Initial research works on the use of glucagon in order to produce colonic hypotony demonstrated that glucagon inhibits all wave activity in the colon [39-41], induces relaxation of the rectosigmoid junction [42], inhibits both electrical and pressure rhythms [43]. This last effect was postulated to be related to a direct action of glucagon on colonic smooth muscles. However, *in vivo* studies on cats led to the assumption that glucagon inhibits the activity of intestinal smooth muscles through the release of catecholamines from the adrenal medulla [44]. Volunteers undergoing barium enema examination reported less discomfort after glucagon than after atropine sulfate [45]. The results of this study were soon confirmed by other investigators [46-48].

In a randomized, double-blind, crossover study on ten healthy adult subjects, and on fifty adults scheduled for barium examination participating in a similar study without crossover, glucagon (2 mg i.m. 10 minutes prior to barium enema) was preferred over placebo by subjects (less discomfort) and by radiologists (more bowel relaxation) [47]. More adverse side effects (nausea, vomiting, headache, abdominal distress) were reported with

glucagon, but the difference did not achieve statistical significance. Pulse and blood pressure were not altered by glucagon. No ECG changes were reported.

Thus, the idea was accepted that glucagon renders the barium enema examination more comfortable, shortens examination times in infants [49] and is a safe drug with only few side effects, such as nausea and vomiting, and few absolute contraindications [50-52]. But soon came the day of reckoning.

Thoeni, Vandeman and Wall [53] undertook a prospective double-blind crossover study in the same patients to determine whether the diagnostic accuracy of double-contrast studies is increased after glucagon (1 mg i.v.) compared with the accuracy after placebo injections. Surprisingly, no significant difference was found between colon hypotony and the quality of examination after glucagon or placebo. Furthermore, glucagon does not significantly improve the sensitivity and specificity of the DCBE examination, although diverticulitis is more accurately diagnosed after glucagon owing to spasm resolution. The Authors recommend "that glucagon be readily available in the fluoroscopy room for double-contrast barium enema examinations but be used only in selected instances". That is: patients with great discomfort during the initial examination, with diffuse or localized spasm or functional colon disorders, with difficulty in retaining the barium, with suspected colitis and diverticulitis. This procedure may justify the high cost of the drug.

Bova, Jurdi and Bennet [54] found no significant differences after glucagon administration (1 mg i.v.) in the degree of colonic distention seen on single- and double-contrast barium enemas, and in the number of patients with focal spasms. Since the colon seems to be less sensitive to glucagon than gastroduodenal segments, the Authors suggest that a different agent should be used to obtain hypotony for more than 20 minutes.

The rate of reflux into the small intestine during the barium enema may increase to 75% with the use of glucagon [34-36]. The older the patient, the more reflux is likely to occur. Glucagon may act to decrease antegrade small intestine peristalsis, relax the ileocecal valve, decrease small intestine intraluminal pressure while leaving colonic intraluminal pressure unaffected [36]. Although barium reflux can supply important additional information on the terminal ileum, retrograde reflux of air into the small intestine lessens colonic distension, sometimes degrading the quality of the examination [55]. From this point of view, routine administration of glucagon during DCBE examination must be considered with caution.

Intracolonic pressure does not change in dogs with or without use of glucagon during a single- or double-contrast barium enema study [56]. In two patients [57] and in seven normal subjects [58] no measurable effect on intraluminal colonic pressure was observed after administration of glucagon. In other reports, no change in intraluminal colonic pressure seemed to accompany glucagon administration [36, 41], while intraluminal pressure in the small intestine decreased significantly [59].

Glucagon has been advocated as the drug of choice to relieve segmental or diffuse colonic spasm [46, 51, 60], but cases may be encountered in which persistent spasm leads to a non diagnostic DCBE examination or erroneously suggests colonic disease [61].

Despite the so much extolled safety of glucagon, the problem has recently been thrust in the limelight again [62-64]. A case of erythema multiforme, the Stevens-Johnson syndrome, after intravenous administration of 0.1 mg glucagon was described by Edell [65]. The possibility of such delayed reactions should be considered and the patient should be alerted.

Three anaphylactic and one allergic reactions occurring during double-contrast studies using glucagon were reported by Gelfand, Sowers, Deponte et al. [66] While the allergic potential of additives in barium suspensions has long been known, the possibility exists of infrequent but occasionally severe allergic and anaphylactic reactions due to glucagon use during gastrointestinal studies. Considering the severity of the reactions, the Authors deem "it prudent to maintain an antiallergic resuscitation kit in the fluoroscopy suite".

Dol and Blom [67] reported the occurrence of a flushing attack after i.v. injection of glucagon prior to double-contrast examination of the stomach, but the patient was subsequently proved to be affected by a carcinoid tumor.

Nausea, abdominal distress, diarrhea, headache, dizziness, dry mouth are reported with significant frequency after i.v. glucagon administration from 0.25 to 2 mg during double-contrast examination of the upper gastrointestinal tract [68]. Reports of nausea increase significantly with glucagon dose increase.

Some remarks should be made on the above mentioned reports. First of all, though glucagon is a naturally occurring hormone in humans, it becomes a proper drug when introduced from outside the body. Therefore, in order to obtain the effects desired with its administration, also unwanted side and adverse effects must be accepted. Well, the administration of an exogenous drug which may sometimes have minor and transient, subjectively felt side effects, may be less dangerous for the patient than an endogenous drug, apparently without side effects, which occasionally may lead to life-threatening adverse effects. In other words, we prefer by far inducing a mydriatic effect every day, in our patients, which wears off in 3 hours and a disturbance of accommodation which does not hamper the possibility to drive a car, than facing a serious unexpected anaphylactic reaction once every two years.

Secondly, glucagon is not routinely administered in DCBE, but selectively in presence of spasm or similar situations. The rationale of hypotonic examination of the colon was well explained by Gohel, Dalinka and Coren [60]: "Significant spasm or narrowing may cause considerable discomfort. If the spasm does not subside with reassurance and temporary cessation of the flow of barium, the patient may evacuate, making it impossible to determine whether the obstruction is organic or functional. Hypotonic examination is most helpful in such cases".

It would appear, however, that the mechanism involved in the antispastic action exerted by glucagon in these situations is different from the mechanism involved in hypotonic induction proper. In case of diffuse or segmental spasm, the number and affinity of accessible adrenergic receptors are assumed to increase significantly, thus leading to an appreciable relaxation which, conversely, is not detectable or is only slightly so in a normally functioning colon. Such indication to the use of glucagon, which has resisted opposing experimental results on the effects of this drug on colon tone and motility, is *per se* a further demonstration that, in science, the empirical observation of an event often precedes its inference based on the theoretical knowledge of the underlying mechanisms.

Spasm during DCBE performance, whether

symptomatic or asymptomatic, is indicative of an abnormal situation which may remain occasional if the radiologist refrains from using too many heavy maneuvers for such an "irritable" organ like the colon. How often does this situation occur in clinical practice? In our experience with the Genoa technique it happens so rarely that the employment of a hypotonic drug, in our opinion, would be absolutely insignificant were it used just to solve situations of this type. Perhaps, the constant, preliminary psychological assistance to the patient, through an open dialogue, whereby the reasons for the examination are carefully explained to the patient is helpful. Perhaps, the bowel preparation regimen, whereby colon functions are not interfered with for 12-15 hours before the examination also helps. Or, perhaps, the easy and fast flow up along the colon, by gravity, of the low density and low viscosity barium suspension in view of its expected *in vivo* thickening because of interaction with magnesium ions is also helpful. Or, perhaps, for other reasons more.

Yet, the fundamental problem is different. Also without any spasm or narrowing, once the colon has been smoothly filled, the use of a hypotonic drug, with its proper physiologic and pharmacological meaning, is precious. The more mucosal surface is available to the radiologist for a detailed analysis, the greater will be the anatomical resolution of the examination: this can be considered the rule of thumb in every DCBE examination. Indeed, one of the basic assumptions in the Welin [69] technique, which is still the gold standard in DCBE performance, is that a properly hypotonic colon which can thus be adequately distended during air insufflation, is "always" fundamental for success.

This means that our aim is to let a functionally normal colon be distended without resistance, which otherwise would set it against itself with subsequent temporary induction of undesired signs of radiologically detectable functional disorders. The block of the autonomic nervous system component in charge of colon tone and motility and of muscarinic cholinergic receptors, is the simplest and most effective way to do so.

From this point of view, glucagon cannot meet the assumptions of a correct preparation to the DCBE examination, since it fails to induce any significant hypotonic action on the colon in normal individuals. Hence, the choice made to date by the Genoa technique (and also by several european institutions) of antimuscarinic drugs. With regard to these drugs, after the introduction of products with a more selective action on the smooth muscles of the gastrointestinal tract - i.e. Buscopan - many past discussions on the side effects of this family of drugs, generally related to the use of atropine (which still plays an important role as pre-anesthetic but is almost totally obsolete in radiology) could be considered overcome.

In agreement with Lee [70], if it is true that situations which may be a contraindication to the use of antimuscarinic drugs or in any case an indication to their careful use occur mainly in the elderly, it is also true that those who have a large experience in the use of these drugs do not have many unpleasant experiences of untoward effects in this class of individuals. So great is our confidence in this drug that we did not feel the need to test other similar drugs or with a different action mechanism.

The "Glucagon case", after all, is not due to a free choice among drugs which exert similar actions on the colon, but rather to a well-reasoned choice of the rationale to be followed in the management of the radiological examination. In our department, our current approach is compulsory hypotony induction, where Buscopan is an integral part of the Genoa technique. The use of glucagon may occasionally be recommended, as clearly indicated in the following questionnaire [71].

A) Have you ever had X-ray of the intestine?   YES   NO

    If YES, what did they find?
    – ulcerative colitis?   1
    – sigmoid diverticulitis?   2

B) Have you taken any medicine in the last two weeks?   YES   NO

    If YES:
    – dicumarol anticoagulants?   3
    – antihistamines?   4
    – Largactil or similar other drug?   5
    – Tofranil or similar other drug?   6

C) Is your blood pressure normal?   YES   NO

    If NO, do you have hypertension bouts?   7

D) Have you ever had an electrocardiogram?   YES   NO

    If YES:
    – myocardial ischemia?   8
    – heart rhythm alterations?   9

    If NO:
    – palpitation?   10

E) Do you suffer from diabetes?   YES   NO
         11

F) Have you ever fainted?
Were you OK again after eating some sugar?   YES   NO
         12

G) Do you have an enlarged prostate?
Do you have difficulty urinating?   YES   NO
         13

H) Do you sometimes have blurred vision?
Do your eyes hurt sometimes?   YES   NO
         14

I) Are you going to drive immediately after the
examination or operate complex machines?   YES   NO
         15

If the reply to question 1 is YES: maximum attention in the use of hypotonic drugs. If there are no specific diagnostic requirements: low pressure SCBE.

If the reply to question 2 is YES glucagon administration prior to the examination may be advisable (if replies to questions 3, 7, 11 and 12 are NO).

If the reply to questions 3, 7, 11 and 12 is YES: be careful in the use of glucagon.

If the reply to questions 4–6, 8–10, and 13–15 is YES : be careful using Buscopan.

References

1. Bilbao MK, Rosch J, Frische LH et al (1968) Hypotonic duodenography in the diagnosis of pancreatic disease. Semin Roentgenol 3:280-287
2. Daniel O, Basu PK, Al-Sumarrae HM (1974) Use of glucagon in the treatment of acute diverticulitis. BMJ 3:720-724
3. Kadir S, Gadacz TR (1987) Adjuncts and modifications to basket retrieval of retained biliary calculi. Cardiovasc Intervent Radiol 10:295-300
4. Ferrucci JT Jr, Long JA Jr (1977) Radiologic treatment of esophageal food impaction using intravenous glucagon. Radiology 125:25-28
5. Trenkner SW, Maglinte DDT, Lehman G et al (1983) Esophageal food impaction: treatment with glucagon. Radiology 149:401-403
6. Fisher JK, Germann DR (1977) Glucagon-aided reduction of intussusception. Radiology 122:197-198
7. Hoy GR, Dunbar D, Boles ET Jr (1977) The use of glucagon in the diagnosis and management of ileocolic intussusception. J Pediatr Surg 12:939-944
8. Haase GM, Boles ET Jr (1979) Glucagon in experimental intussusception. J Pediatr Surg 14:664-669
9. Franken EA Jr, Smith W, Chernish SM et al (1983) The use of glucagon in hydrostatic reduction of intussusception. A double-blind study of 30 patients. Radiology 146:687
10. Mortensson W, Eklof O, Laurin S (1984) Hydrostatic reduction of childhood intussusception. The role of adjuvant glucagon medication. Acta Radiol (Diagn) 25:261-264
11. Berstock DA, Wood JR, Williams R (1982) The glucagon test in obstructive and hepatocellular jaundice. Postgrad Med J 58:485-486
12. Kreel L (1975) Pharmaco-radiology in barium examinations with special reference to glucagon. Br J Radiol 48:691-703
13. Kreel L (1979) Glucagon in radiology - A review. Australas Radiol 23:202-208
14. Thoeni RF, Margulis AR (1988) The state of radiographic technique in the examination of the colon: A survey in 1987. Radiology 167:7-12
15. Mojsov SG, Heinrich G, Wilson IB et al (1986) Preproglucagon gene expression in pancreas and intestine diversifies at the level of post-transcriptional processing. J Biol Chem 261:11880-11889
16. Peterson DR, Carone FA, Oparil S et al (1982) Differences between renal tubular processing of glucagon and insulin. Am J Physiol 242:F112-F118
17. Lawrence AM (1967) Glucagon provocative test for pheochromocytoma. Ann Intern Med 66:1091-1096
18. Lefebvre PJ, Cession-Fossion AM, Luyckx AS (1968) Interrelationships glucagon-adrenergic system in experimental and clinical conditions. Arch Int Pharmacodyn Ther 172:393-404
19. Lawrence AM (1969) Glucagon. Annu Rev Med 20:207-223
20. Thorell JI, Person B (1970) Side-effects of insulin contaminating commercial glucagon (letter). Lancet 2:52-53
21. Kitabchi AE, Lamkin N Jr, Lieberman P et al (1975) Allergic response to glucagon injection as a result of insulin contamination. J Clin Endocrinol Metab 41:863-867
22. Physicians' desk reference (1987) 41st ed. Oradell, NJ: Medical Economics, pp 1141-1142
23. Lawrence AM (1969) Glucagon. Annu Rev Med 20:207-223
24. Dreiling DA, Janowitz HD (1959) Effect of glucagon on gastric secretion in man. Gastroenterology 36:580-581
25. Necheles H, Sparn J, Walker L (1966) Effect of glucagon on gastrointestinal motility. Am J Gastroenterol 45:29-34
26. Dyck WP, Janowitz HD (1971) Effect of glucagon on hepatic bile secretion in man. Gastroenterology 60:400-404
27. Jones RS, Hall AD (1969) Effect of glucagon on Brunner's gland secretion in dogs. Proc Soc Exp Biol Med 132:1151-1159
28. Chernish SM, Miller SE, Rosenak BD et al (1972) Hypotonic duodenography with the use of glucagon. Gastroenterology 63:392-398
29. Miller RE, Chernish SM, Rosenak BD et al (1973) Hypotonic duodenography with glucagon. Radiology 108:35-42
30. Miller RE, Chernish SM, Skucas J et al (1974) Hypotonic roentgenography with glucagon. AJR 121:264-274.
31. Carsen GM, Finby N (1976) Hypotonic duodenography with glucagon: A clinical comparison study. Radiology 118:529-533
32. Bertrand G, Linscheer WG, Raheja KL et al (1977) Double-blind evaluation of glucagon and propantheline bromide (pro-banthine) for hypotonic duodenography. AJR 128:197-200
33. Hogan WJ, Dodds WJ, Hoke SE et al (1975) Effect of glucagon on esophageal motor function. Gastroenterology 69:160-165
34. Hage G (1974) Méthode rapide de radiographie du colon en double contrast: utilisation du glucagon. Arch Fr Mal App Dig 63:297-303
35. Violon D, Steppe R, Potvliege R (1981) Improved retrograde ileography with glucagon. AJR 136:833-834
36. Monsein LH, Halpert RD, Harris ED et al (1986) Retrograde ileography: Value of glucagon. Radiology 161:558-559
37. Rothe AJ, Young JWR, Kermati B (1987) The value of glucagon in routine barium investigations of the gastrointestinal tract. Invest Radiol 22:786-791
38. Paul F, Freyschmidt J (1976) The use of glucagon for endoscopic and radiological examination of the gastrointestinal tract. Fortschr Geb Rontgenstr Nuklearmed 125:31-37
39. Chowdhury AR, Lorber SH (1974) Effects of glucagon and secretion on food or morphine induced motor activity of the distal colon, rectum and anal sphincter (abstract). Am Fed Clin Res 22:693
40. Chowdhury AR, Dinoso V, Lorber SH (1976) Characterization of hyperactive segment of the rectosigmoid junction. Gastroenterology 71:584-588
41. Chowdhury AR, Lorber SH (1977) Effects of glucagon and secretion on food or morphine induced motor activity of the distal colon, rectum and anal sphincter. Am J Dig Dis 22:775-780
42. Paul F (1974) Quantitative studies of the effect of pancreatic glucagon and secretin on gastrointestinal motility in man recorded by simultaneous electromanometric registration. Klin Wochenschr 52:983-989

43. Taylor I, Duthie HL, Cumberland DC et al (1975) Glucagon and the colon. Gut 16:973-978

44. Fasth S, Hulten L (1971) Effect of glucagon on intestinal motility and blood flow. Acta Physiol Scand 83:169-173

45. Miller RE, Chernish SM, Skucas J et al (1974) Hypotonic colon examination with glucagon. Radiology 113:555-562

46. Meeroff JC, Jorgens J, Isenberg JI (1975) The effect of glucagon on barium enema examination. Radiology 115:5-7

47. Harned RK, Stelling CB, Williams S et al (1976) Glucagon and barium enema examinations: A controlled clinical trial. AJR 126:981-984

48. Munro TG (1979) Pitfalls to avoid: spasm in ulcerative colitis masquerading as carcinoma. J Can Assoc Radiol 30:171-172

49. Ratcliffe JF (1980) Glucagon in barium examinations in infants and children: special reference to dosage. Br J Radiol 53:860-862

50. Jerele JJ (1976) Use of glucagon as the hypotonic agent in barium enema examination. J Am Osteopath Assoc 76:264-271

51. Miller RE, Chernish SM, Brunelle RL (1976) Gastrointestinal radiology with glucagon. Gastrointest Radiol 4:1-10

52. Miller RE, Chernish SM (1981) On the use of glucagon - Ancillary effects and other considerations. In: Picazo J (ed) Gastroenterology and hepatology. Pharmacological, clinical, and therapeutic implications. Lancaster, England: MTP Press, pp 57-66

53. Thoeni RF, Vandeman F, Wall SD (1984) Effect of glucagon on the diagnostic accuracy of double-contrast barium enema examinations. AJR 142:111-114

54. Bova JG, Jurdi RA, Bennett WF (1993) Antispasmodic drugs to reduce discomfort and colonic spasm during barium enemas: Comparison of oral hyoscyamine, IV glucagon, and no drug. AJR 161:965-968

55. Stone EE, Conte FA (1988) Glucagon-induced small bowel air reflux: Degradating effects on double-contrast colon examination. Gastrointest Radiol 13:212-214

56. Thoeni RF, Margulis AR (1979) Intracolonic pressures during barium enema studies using the single- and double-contrast techniques. Invest Radiol 14:162-165

57. Diner WC, Patel G, Texter EC et al (1981) Intraluminal pressure measurements during barium enema: full column vs. air contrast. AJR 137:217-221

58. Oliva L, Cittadini G (1981) Il clisma a doppio contrasto: problemi metodologici e tecnici. Verona: Cortina

59. Patel GK, Whalen GE, Soergel KH et al (1979) Glucagon effect on the human small intestine. Am J Dig Dis 24:501-508

60. Gohel VK, Dalinka MK, Coren GS (1975) Hypotonic examination of the colon with glucagon. Radiology 115:1-4

61. Levine MS, Gasparaitis AE (1986) Barium filling for glucagon-resistant spasm on double-contrast barium enema examinations. Radiology 160:264-265

62. Hall FM (1987) Pharmacologic agents in gastrointestinal radiology (letter). Radiology 165:289

63. Chernish SM, Maglinte DDT, Brunelle RL (1988) The laboratory response to glucagon dosages used in gastrointestinal examinations. Invest Radiol 23:847-852

64. Chernish SM, Maglinte DDT (1990) Glucagon: common untoward reactions - review and recommendations. Radiology 177:145-146

65. Edell SL (1980) Erythema multiforme secondary to intravenous glucagon. AJR 134:385-386

66. Gelfand DW, Sowers JC, DePonte KA et al (1985) Anaphylactic and allergic reactions during double-contrast studies: Is glucagon or barium suspension the allergen? AJR 144:405-406

67. Dol JA, Blom JMH (1987) A carcinoid flushing attack after intravenous glucagon: A case report. J Med Imaging 1:342-343

68. Miller RE, Chernish SM, Brunelle RL et al (1978) Double-blind radiographic study of dose response to intravenous glucagon for hypotonic duodenography. Radiology 127:55-59

69. Welin S, Welin G (1976) The double contrast examination of the colon. Experience with the Welin modification. Stuttgart: Thieme

70. Lee JR (1982) Routine use of hyoscine N-butylbromide (Buscopan) in double contrast barium enema examinations. Clin Radiol 33:273-276

71. Cittadini G, De Cata T, Giribaldi M (1978) Ipotonizziamo il colon (ma con giudizio). Il Radiologo 17(5):42-44

14 Barium suspensions

Since as early as 1910 [1], barium sulfate and gastrointestinal radiology have been joined together in an indissoluble relationship, while any other alternative contrast materials, like barium metatitanate [2], have failed to replace barium sulfate. As known, the use of iodine-containing water-soluble contrast agents applies only to situations where barium sulfate is contraindicated. The reasons for all this are to be looked for in the *favorable electronic environment of the Ba atom*, which has a good X-photon absorption in the energy range used in roentgendiagnostics, and also in the *excellent tolerance to barium sulfate*, which flows across the intestinal lumen with very little absorption [3,4] and which may raise problems only in case of tight stenosis or perforation [5-8].

The properties of currently available $BaSO_4$ formulations are much different from those available in the past when the compound was supplied as pure powder to be mixed on the spot, purified of any soluble salts in compliance with strict Pharmacopeia rules, and in particular of $BaCl_2$, a highly toxic and contracture producing agent [9]. Using pure $BaSO_4$ suspensions, both *in vitro* and *in vivo*, the disperse phase tends to become separated from the continuous phase, thus the suspension tends to sediment and flocculate, the quality of the intestinal mucosa coating is poor, and it is difficult to achieve the concentration required for certain uses. All these defects are no longer troubling modern preparations, all of which have special formulations designed to increase the quality of intestinal mucosa coating.

Though several attempts have been made to further improve these preparations [10], the products supplied by pharmaceutical industries have often been accepted too passively and lazily by radiologists [11], probably because they trust the relatively safe route - oral and rectal - of barium administration. This is further confirmed by the utterly different involvement in the discussion on water-soluble iodinated contrast media, spurred by a great attention for the route of administration (directly into the blood stream), but also by the dreaded minor and major adverse effects requiring prompt and well targeted therapies. The reasons for some modifications to the initial barium sulfate formulations will be only briefly discussed in this chapter. For a more detailed treatment of this topic, reference should be made to more exhaustive treatises [12].

Barium suspensions and their properties

With barium suspensions prepared on the spot from dry bulk powder barium sulfate, there are no doubts about the chemical composition of the *disperse phase* (100% pure $BaSO_4$) and the *continuous phase* (distilled water or, more commonly, tap water). $BaSO_4$ is supplied in the form of powder consisting of individual particles ranging from approximately 1 to 10 µm, with an average size of 2.5 µm. In general, particle size is not homogeneous, with some prevalence of smaller particles. Each particle contains several thousands of rhombic, four-molecule elementary crystals of about 0.001 µm size. Barium particles are 4.5 times heavier than water, at equal volume: this is *per se* a condition favoring a strong sedimentation of aqueous barium sulfate suspensions.

The particle surface is irregular, featuring proper active spots where other substances present in or purposely added to the solutions (from which crystals are precipitated in industrial barium preparation) tend to be adsorbed. This adsorption may even alter the fundamental structure of the crystal lattice. Adsorbed substances (i.e. organic molecules, organic ions and salts) may be moved due to pH variations. Hence, barium particles, while flowing through the alimentary canal, where pH ranges from intense gastric acidity to the alkaline environment of the other segments, are likely to undergo significant chemical and physicochemical modifications.

$BaSO_4$ molecular weight is 233 atomic mass units, 137 of which, corresponding to 59%, are due to Ba atom. X-photon absorption is the barium sulfate property which is exploited in roentgenology: this property is almost totally due to the Ba atom. Conversely, the whole molecule is responsible for its physicochemical properties which are drastically affected by the presence of any organic or inorganic additives.

The maximum concentration for $BaSO_4$ aqueous solutions is 0.0002 g%: therefore, it is practically insoluble in water. If particles with less than 0.1 µm diameter are used, very diluted, almost transparent solutions can be obtained. Thus, aqueous suspensions are the only pharmaceutical preparations obtainable with a suitable concentration for the radiological use.

The concentration of barium suspensions is generally expressed in $BaSO_4$ grams contained in 100 ml of suspension (weight/volume, or w/v, g% ml); less commonly it is expressed in $BaSO_4$ grams contained in 100 grams of suspension (weight/weight, or w/w, g% g). This latter measurement can be transformed into the former one by multiplying its numerical value by the specific gravity of the suspension. For example, if 1 ml of a 60% w/w barium suspension has a weight of 1.85 g, that is to say its specific gravity is 1.85, the w/v concentration is 111 g% ml. In radiological applications, high concentrations are preferred in order to achieve high radiopacity levels with small suspension volumes.

Viscosity is the physical property of fluids that determines the internal resistance to shear forces. It depends on the amount of internal holding forces (cohesion) versus the attractive force exerted by any external bonds (adhesion). It is normally measured in centipoise (cP) or centistokes (cSt): the cP value equals the cSt value times specific gravity.

Barium suspensions can be considered *newtonian fluids* (namely fluids which, for the absolutely free mutual molecular movements, are characterized by constant viscosity independently of the acting force per surface unit, i.e. shear force) only at low concentrations, below 40% w/w. Conversely, at higher concentrations, they behave like *pseudoplastic fluids*, where viscosity decreases with increasing shear force. This is due to the fact that molecules in resting position take up a mutually disorderly arrangement and align along the fluid motion direction only under the effect of the force acting on them.

Obviously enough, this behaviour is even more evident in modern barium suspensions where compounds are added to increase linear viscosity, such as carboxymethylcellulose or gum ghatti. In this case, in addition to pseudoplastic properties, also another phenomenon can be observed, known as *thixotropy*: viscosity values experimentally obtained by progressively reducing the shear force are different from those obtained by progressively increasing it. This is due to the fact that resting molecules form a three-dimensional mesh with a gel-like texture which breaks when the fluid is subjected to mechanical stress. When left standing, the mesh is slowly formed again thus leading to thixotropy.

In practice, thixotropy is used to increase the stability of barium suspensions: when left standing, they have a good consistency without sedimentation; when shaken, their viscosity rapidly decreases and the material becomes properly fluid. This is the case particularly with Barotrast, a barium suspension used for the double-contrast study of the large bowel, which requires to be strongly shaken with a blender to obtain the suspension for proper use.

When suspended, each particle surface adsorbs water molecules and OH^- ions. Imbibition water molecules, specially in the most internal layers, align in a regular fashion following their bipolar structure. This aqueous cap remarkably reduces particle sedimentation. OH^- ions, due to electrostatic repulsion among the various particles, reduce their tendency to aggregate and flocculate. The adsorption of imbibition water takes place at the surface. Therefore, the greater is the total surface of barium particles in a certain suspension volume (namely the greater is the barium/water interface), the more water will be taken from the continuous phase with subsequent increase in suspension viscosity. Viceversa, the smaller the barium/water interface, the greater the alternative adsorption of OH^- ions, with subsequent increase in suspension fluidity. It can be demonstrated that, at equal barium weight, the total surface of particles increases 10 folds when their diameter is reduced from 10 to 1μm, 20 folds with their reduction to 0.5 μm. Hence, as we shall also see below, the stability and certain physicochemical properties of the barium suspension are affected by particle size.

In practice, by using a pure $BaSO_4$ suspension in water the following problems are likely to arise: suspension sedimentation, spontaneous flocculation, *in vivo* provoked flocculation, segmentation of the barium column in the intestinal lumen, foam formation, poor adhesion to intestinal mucosae, difficulty to obtain sufficiently concentrated suspensions, all of which are of great impact on double-contrast studies. In order to better understand all modern modifications to the suspensions, all these phenomena deserve a more detailed explanation.

Sedimentation

Sedimentation is the progressive separation, under the effect of gravity, of the disperse phase (which deposits on the bottom) from the continuous phase. According to Stokes' law, the sedimentation rate is directly proportional to the specific gravity difference between the two phases and to the square of the diameter of disperse particles, and inversely proportional to the viscosity of the continuous phase.

Therefore, the sedimentation rate can be reduced by decreasing the average diameter of barium particles (*micronization*) or by increasing the viscosity of the suspending medium (*colloidization*). As mentioned above, just by reducing the average diameter of barium particles, a global increase in total suspension viscosity can be obtained but, through the resulting reduction of the alternative OH^- adsorption, electrostatic repulsion of barium particles, which contributes to controlling aggregation and flocculation, is lowered.

Chemical flocculation

Chemical flocculation is the progressive aggregation of barium particles in the form of flocks of a few millimeter size, which are being deposited in accordance to Stokes' law. It results from continuous clashes of dispersed particles, caused by temperature differences inside the suspension and the obvious mechanical stress it is subjected to. It is enhanced by the difference in barium particle size, since larger particles act as *attraction clusters* for smaller ones. It is hampered by electric charges on particle surface inducing electrostatic repulsion among them.

The reduction in the average diameter of barium particles, though useful to limit sedimentation, is detrimental for flocculation control since it promotes the formation of an imbibition H_2O molecule cap at the expense of OH^- ion adsorption. When trying to correct the suspension, a balance is reached with particles of about 1μm diameter. Conversely, an increase in suspension viscosity, since inner particle movements are thus reduced, has a positive impact on controlling chemical flocculation.

With the removal of larger particles and a greater uniformity in their size, which can be obtained during the preparation by precipitation of barium sulfate, chemical flocculation is reduced both *in vivo* and *in vitro*. With this modification, however, the adhesion of barium particles to the intestinal mucosae is slightly reduced.

Biochemical flocculation

In vivo, the attraction clusters of barium particles consist of protein and colloidal glycoprotein polymers which are present in intestinal secretions. These polymers have different electrical behavior depending on the pH of the medium. In the stomach, for example, where pH is strongly acid, they have a positive surface charge. In the other intestinal segments, where pH is more alkaline, they have a negative surface charge. In acid media, they act as real attraction clusters, based on their electrostatic charge, of barium particles, thus promoting flocculation. At the same time, they are an obstacle to the adhesion of barium to the mucosa, hence reducing coating quality. This phenomenon can be easily demonstrated *in vitro* by adding a certain amount of gastric juice to a pure $BaSO_4$ suspension: flocculation increases proportionally up to a saturation level. In this case, mucines play a fundamental role.

Biochemical flocculation is hampered by the increase in the electronegative charge of barium particles. Another important element is the increase in the number of barium particles by volume unit of the suspension, hence its concentration. However, this increase is affected by global viscosity: when viscosity is too high, "pastes" are obtained which, lacking the necessary fluidity, fail to adhere to intestinal mucosae.

Therefore, with regard to flocculation, the use of barium particles that are too small is a disadvantage. Conversely, some increase in suspension viscosity may be helpful as long as it does not affect the suspension concentration obtainable. As mentioned above, by reducing the number of larger particles, biochemical flocculation is diminished.

Barium column segmentation

This phenomenon, which is mostly evident in the small bowel, is to be attributed to a poor miscibility of the barium suspension with intestinal secretions. The slower is the suspension transit in the intestine, the more intense barium column segmentation will be. In fact, segmentation is avoided by adding water repellent and surface-active agents to the barium suspension which promote its uniform blending with intestinal secretions, and also by adding substances speeding up its transit (for example sorbitol).

Adhesion to intestinal mucosae

The weakness of conventional barium suspensions is that a good coating of intestinal mucosa, though fundamental in mucosal relief evaluation and high resolution double-contrast study, is successfully achieved only occasionally.

For an optimal coating, the barium film has to meet the following conditions: cover the mucosa by following its relief in a homogeneous way, without cracks, in a sufficiently thin layer so as not to hide any normal or pathological findings (thus, of maximum a few hundreds μm thickness), must be stable in time, have good breaking strength to withstand the dynamic effects of intestinal movements (therefore, with a good surface tension), and be adequately radiopaque (thus, with high density).

The mechanisms by which a film with the features described above can actually be obtained and the various factors affecting such features are still the object of several speculations based on physicochemical and biochemical assumptions which, in most cases, can be proved or disproved only through radiological examination experience [3]. The very fact that even with pure $BaSO_4$ suspensions in water some mucosal coating is indeed achieved, is already evidence that barium particles alone can adhere to the mucosa. The instability of the suspension due to unsuitable physicochemical properties is the main responsible for the irregular and variable nature of such event. Theoretically speaking, this adhesion could be compared to a kind of micro-sedimentation micro-flocculation of barium particles under the effects of the following two mechanisms: *adsorption of barium particles on mucoproteinic and glycoproteinic colloids* covering the mucosal surface like a veil; *electrostatic attraction of barium particles with a negative surface charge.*

The most favorable condition for barium particle adhesion would be the total absence of intestinal secretions, something which, to some extent, can be achieved in the colon with anticholinergic drugs (atropine, for example), but not so feasible at gastric level because of the extreme pH conditions and, hence, the need for an adequate protection against flocculation. In practice, the best one can do is to promote miscibility of the barium suspension with intestinal secretions by adding surfactant agents, containing hydrophilic and lyophilic groups by which, through proper molecule orientation, interface tension is reduced and, therefore, miscibility enhanced. As already mentioned before, the concurrent increase in the number of negatively charged barium particles to oppose flocculation caused by the neutralization of the small charge present there, is also particularly beneficial.

The use of surfactants has long been tested by radiologists, such as some types of tween, sodium lauryl sulfate, saponins, which greatly improve miscibility as theoretically expected. However, at the same time, they induce the formation of foam which may be particularly annoying in the examination of mucosa details [14].

The real impact of electrostatic attraction can be verified by studying mucosal coating quality with barium particles having different average diameters. According to what stated above, when the average diameter of barium particles decreases, imbibition water adsorption increases with subsequent reduction in the adsorption of alternative OH^- ions. The average diameter reduction of particles in micronized preparations has a favorable impact on mucosal coating because the suspension becomes more stable. However, in order to let the factors favoring coating quality (greater suspension stability, increased viscosity) prevail over those which are detrimental to it (expected reduction in negative surface charges), a heavy use of *colloidal additives* is required with many accessible negatively charged groups to protect and "glue" together the barium particles and the mucosa. Such a condition is reversed around 0.5-0.8 μm, below which value no further micronization is advisable.

When large sized barium particles are used - which has empirically proved to be beneficial in double-contrast studies of the upper digestive tract - practically perfect coating is achieved without viscosity-enhancing and colloidal additives, but only with *peptizing additives* (sodium citrate, whose effect seems to be enhanced by sorbitol, is the most active one). Inducing the release of imbibition water after the masking of strongly hydrophilic SO_4^{--} ions by less hydrophilic citrate ions seems to be their exclusive function. Hence, the greater amount of free water available allows to obtain extremely high $BaSO_4$ concentrations (with E-Z-HD, having 20 μm diameter particles, up to 250% w/v concentrations can be obtained).

Many additives used for protection-stabilization purposes in modern barium suspensions establish very close physical and physicochemical relations with barium particles: in some cases they are added as desired impurities to the solution from which, during preparation, barium sulfate particles are precipitated, in other cases they are added later, in dry form, or also directly to the suspension.

Lyophobic colloids coat barium particles through adsorption inducing the formation of a double envelope of electric charges. These charges, which can be neutralized under extreme pH conditions or in the presence of surplus electrolytes, counteract the flocculation of particles through electrostatic repulsion and, at the same time, favor electrostatic adhesion to the mucosal surface.

Lyophilic colloids coat the particle either directly or through the already coated particle by the lyophobic colloid supplying it with a great amount of imbibition water. They are thus active as viscosity-enhancing and protective additives. The high number of ionic groups in their linear structure

and in the lateral groups significantly promotes the adhesion of the coated particle to the mucosal surface through a proper gluing mechanism. For this reason they are correctly called *gums*.

In some cases, they are natural products (such as gum ghatti, which is one of the main additives of Polibar ACB). In other cases they are synthetic, easily processable products with good viscosity-enhancing, gluing properties and resistance against bacterial attack (see carboxymethylcellulose, which is one of the main additives of Barotrast). To make these gums soluble is, from a practical point of view, a difficult job: the gum ghatti undergoes aquation, its linear chain is broken into smaller fragments and, after addition of water, the desired result is obtained just with normal manual shaking. Conversely, carboxymethylcellulose needs to be mechanically shaken to induce the extempore breaking of its chain. Gum selection is essential in the planning of a good barium contrast medium, since it has a direct impact on the gluing power and hence on the coating quality of the mucosa, which is a fundamental feature in the implementation of modern double-contrast techniques. The nature of the gum and the length of its chain play an important role.

Obviously enough, the ideal film thickness is the minimum allowable, compatibly with sufficient radiopacity. Since radiopacity is directly proportional to barium sulfate concentration, the advantage of using suspensions with a high specific gravity (hence with a high Ba atoms concentration) and low viscosity (which is necessary to obtain high Ba concentrations) is self-evident. At equal thickness, radiological density, and therefore X-ray absorption, increases 1.8 times from a 43% w/w to a 60% w/w barium suspension, and 2.5 times from a 33% w/w to a 60% w/w one [11]. Or, which means practically the same, radiopacity remains the same with a 1.8 or 2.5 times thinner film. It is thus important to obtain suspensions which are stable at high concentration.

By increasing suspension viscosity, namely reducing its fluidity - i.e. its tendency to move on - mucosal adhesion is enhanced. Radiological practice has indeed shown a direct proportion between viscosity and film thickness. This is true up to a certain point, beyond which the negative effects are felt due to lower miscibility with intestinal secretions, lower concentrations achievable, excessively slow transit in the intestine.

A sufficient surface tension must be maintained in order to ensure barium film resistance, that is to say to maintain film uniformity but also to level out any cracks in its weakest points (air bubbles, mucus build-up, small flock clusters, mechanic cracks caused by intestinal movements). However, if surface tension is too high, the film may wrinkle, thus creating radiologically demonstrated artifacts.

In radiological practice, film thickness and features also depend on personal preferences and habits of the radiologist. In disputes among supporters of the various barium preparations, it is difficult to take an objective position, since it never happens in practice that a diagnosis made with one type fails with another one for lack of anatomic resolution.

Foam formation

Formation of foam is a nuisance in the double-contrast study of the digestive tract since artifacts can be produced which may sometimes be difficult to distinguish from pathologic findings (for example, in DCBE, an air bubble can be mistaken for a polyp). The general theory on foam formation is very complex and there are still doubts on the various factors involved in this event. In fact, many *a priori* judgments on the foaminess of a solution are often disproved by practice.

The tendency to foam formation is increased when the interface tension of the barium suspension is reduced, something which is required to improve suspension stability as well as its miscibility with intestinal secretions, penetration into mucosal recesses and perhaps also adhesiveness. Barium particles alone, through a floating mechanism, stabilize the foam by arranging themselves between the individual bubbles. Lyophobic colloids prevent foam formation, while lyophilic ones enhance it. Viscous suspensions form less foam. Electric charges stabilize the foam: from this point of view, the addition of pH neutralizing electrolytes remarkably reduces foam formation. The type of water is also important since, in principle, foam formation is reduced by hard water which, on the other side, can precipitate additives which are important for suspension stability. From all this it is clear that corrections sometimes may worsen the original suspension characteristics: for example, paradoxically enough, by the addition of highly lypophilic

and poorly hydrophilic surfactants (silicon compounds) which *per se* can induce sedimentation.

*

What has been described so far can be briefly summarized in the following few statements:

1. It is practically impossible to obtain pure barium sulfate suspensions in water with the stability and properties required by modern gastrointestinal radiology.
2. Several defects already detected *in vitro* are worsened *in vivo*.
3. Modifications of various types are possible: however, due to interconnected instability factors, by correcting one defect another may be worsened.
4. Due to different environments in the various intestinal segments, specially with reference to the type of secretion and pH, it is impossible to obtain one single barium suspension by which all the different conditions present in the various segments can be properly met at the same time.
5. In principle, specific formulations are required for the double-contrast study of the stomach and the colon. For the esophagus, "stomach type" barium suspensions are suitable, whereas for the study of the small intestine through jejunal intubation, "colon type" barium suspensions are suitable.
6. Fundamentally, all the possible corrections boil down to the following two modifications: optimization of barium sulfate particle size; addition to the suspending medium of additives, many of them colloidals.
7. A precise indication from the industry is necessary, not so much with regard to the technological preparation process of the product, no matter whether it comes in powder or lyophilized preparation or in a ready-to-use suspension, but especially with reference to all the substances present and related quantities. It is important to evaluate all possible allergies to these substances [15-18], or any interference with the laboratory examinations that the patient may undergo concurrently with the radiological examination.

The analysis presented here is important, because it allows the radiologist to be aware of the multiple factors involved in the formulation of a barium suspension suitable to meet modern radiological needs, and to be able to duly assess such factors, should he deem it proper to make some personal corrections. In Table 1, some physicochemical features are indicated

Tabella 1. Some radiologically significant physicochemical properties of the most commonly used barium suspensions

Suspension	Concentration (% w/v)	pH	Density (g/cm³)	Viscosity (cSt at 20°C)
Polibar ACB (Prontobario Colon)	100	6.5	1.77	63
	75		1.51	21.4
	50		1.31	7.3
	25		1.19	2.9
Mixobar 70 DC	70	4.1	1.40	95
	50		1.30	33.5
	35		1.17	13.7
	25		1.08	6.1
Barotrast	50	7.8	1.39	147.3
	35		1.25	43.3
	25		1.18	18.5
	17.5		1.13	9.2
Micropaque	100	4.3	1.67	69.7
	75		1.43	22.7
	50		1.26	8.7
	25		1.19	3.1
E-Z-HD (Prontobario HD)	250	6.5	2.80	357.1

of the barium suspensions most commonly used in the double-contrast examination of the colon.

With regard to DCBE, it should be noted that the exclusive function of the radiotransparent gaseous contrast medium employed is to distend the intestinal lumen after completion of barium mucosal coating. The type of gas employed is important not so much for possible interactions with the barium coating, but rather because it may affect the patient's tolerance for the examination. For example, CO_2, which is reabsorbed by the colonic mucosa more rapidly than air [19], is preferred by some Authors [20-22]. Yet, it would not appear to have acquired great support [23-25].

References

1. Bachem C, Günther H (1910) Bariumsulfat als schattenbildendes Kontrastmittel bei Röntgenuntersuchungen. Zeitschr Rontgenkunde Rad Forschr 12:369-376
2. Heitz F, Heitz L (1974) Presentation d'un nouveau produit de contraste en radiologie digestive: le titanate de baryum. J Radiol Electrol Med Nucl 55:430-431
3. Mauras Y, Allain P, Roques MA et al (1983) Étude de l'absorption digestive du baryum après l'administration orale du sulfate de baryum pour exploration radiologique. Thérapie 38:109-110
4. Clavel JP, Lorillot ML, Buthiau D et al (1987) Absorption intestinale du baryum lors de l'explorations radiologiques. Thérapie 42:239-243
5. Zheutlin N, Lasser EC, Rigler LG (1952) Clinical studies on effect of barium in the peritoneal cavity following rupture of the colon. Surgery 32:967-979
6. Westfall RH, Nelson RH, Musselman MM (1966) Barium peritonitis. Am J Surg 112:760-763
7. Masel H, Masel JP, Casey KV (1971) A survey of colon examination techniques in Australia and New Zealand, with a review of complications. Australas Radiol 15:140-147
8. Miller RE, Skucas J, Violante MR et al (1975) The effect of barium on blood in the gastrointestinal tract. Radiology 117:527-530
9. Amberg JR, Unger JD (1970) Contamination of barium sulfate suspension. Radiology 97:182-183
10. Miller RE (1965) Barium Sulfate Suspensions. Radiology 84:241-251
11. Brown GR (1963) High-density barium-sulfate suspensions: an improved diagnostic medium. Radiology 81: 839-845
12. Skucas J (1989) Radiographic contrast agents. Second Edition. Rockville, Maryland: Aspen
13. Cittadini G (1979) Bario senza veli. Il Radiologo 18 (4): 32-39
14. Embring G, Mattsson O (1968) Barium Contrast Agents. Acta Radiol (Diagn) 7: 245-256
15. Schwartz EE, Glick SN, Foggs MB et al (1984) Hypersensitivity reactions after barium enema examination. AJR 143:103-104

16. McAvoy M, Young JWR, Keramati B (1985) Hypersensitivity reactions to barium suspension (letter). AJR 144:1316

17. Gelfand DW, Sowers JC, DePonte KA et al (1985) Anaphylactic and allergic reactions during double-contrast studies: is glucagon or barium suspension the allergen? AJR 144:405-406

18. Janower ML (1986) Hypersensitivity reactions after barium studies of the upper and lower gastrointestinal tract. Radiology 161:139-140

19. Levene G (1957) Rates of venous absorption of carbon dioxide and air used in double-contrast examination of the colon. Radiology 69:571-575

20. Coblenz CL, Frost RA, Molinaro V et al (1985) Pain after barium enema: effect of CO_2 and air on double-contrast study. Radiology 157:35-36

21. Bassette JR, Maglinte DDT (1987) Double-contrast barium enema study: simple conversion to CO_2. Radiology 162:274-275

22. Bernier P, Coblentz C (1986) CO_2 delivery system for double-contrast barium enema examinations. Radiology 159:264

23. Scullion DA, Wetton CW, Davies C et al (1995) The use of air or CO_2 as insufflation agents for double contrast barium enema (DCBE): is there a qualitative difference? Clin Radiol 50:558-561

24. Skovgaard N, Sloth C, von Benzon E et al (1995) The role of carbon dioxide and atmospheric air in double-contrast barium enema. Abdom Imaging 20:436-439

25. Farrow R, Jones AMM, Wallace DA et al (1995) Air versus carbon dioxide insufflation in double contrast barium enemas: the role of active gaseous drainage. Br J Radiol 68:838-840

15 Which barium suspension?

As demonstrated by practice, there is some interdependence between the various phases in DCBE implementation. For example, better results can be obtained either with a higher or a lower viscosity and density barium suspensions depending on the selected protocol for bowel preparation, which leaves the colonic mucosa in a more or less hydrated condition. Also, depending on the desired mucosal coating contrast, a high or, respectively, medium kilovoltage radiographic technique is likely to yield better results. Therefore, the type of barium suspension is a decisive factor for the determination of the final results.

In Italy, since 1987, about 440,000 barium enema examinations are carried out every year [1], of which slightly more than 60% apply the double-contrast technique. Though other barium sulfate formulations and various blends of different preparations have been extensively tested [2], currently only three different proprietary formulations are mostly used which have been specifically designed for the double-contrast examination of the colon:

• Polibar ACB (E-Z-EM, Westbury, NY), supplied under the brand name of Prontobario Colon (Bracco, Milan), by far the most popular one, a micronized 94% w/w barium sulfate formulation containing gum ghatti, sodium citrate, sodium carrageenan, sorbitol, simethicone, polyoxyethylene glyceryl mono-oleate, available in a vinyl bag with snap-cap, prefilled with 400 grams of powder. It is worth noting that with the Polibar formulation available in Italy, probably because of a different nature and concentration of the added gum, the suspension obtainable is slightly different in pH, density and viscosity from Polibar in the United States (see Table 1 in Chap. 14).

• Mixobar 70% D.C. and more recently Mixobar 100% (Byk Gulden Italia, Cormano, Milan), a very practical and stable formulation supplied in the form of a ready-to-use 70% or 100% w/v barium sulfate suspension containing gum xanthan (Keltrol), citric acid, potassium sorbate, simethicone, sodium salt of polyalkylnaphthalene sulfonic acid, methyl-p-hydroxybenzoate;

• Barotrast (Barnes Hind, Sunnyvale, California), distributed by Benco, Rome, a micronized 92.5% w/w barium sulfate formulation containing carboxymethylcellulose, bentonite, sodium saccharin, available in form of powder with a measuring cup for proper dosage.

Our experience mainly refers, successfully, to these formulations. A special attention was drawn in the initial steps of the Genoa technique to Barotrast and Polibar ACB, two products with many differential features (Table 1), which, after the detailed analysis of Chapter 14, will be mentioned only briefly.

The selection of the gum used as viscosity-enhancing agent is very important. Natural gums (pectins, gum ghatti) or artificial ones (carboxymethylcellulose), maintain the barium in disperse phase and facilitate its contact with the mucosa by increasing surface tension and through thixotropy. These gums consist of a long colloidal polymer chain, which may need a strong shaking to be sus-

Table 1. Differential features between Barotrast and Polibar ACB

Barotrast
suspended only after intense shaking with blender
tannic acid is tolerated
pressure injector is required for administration
colon emptying difficult to perform
formation of air bubbles
moderate air/barium levels
thick coating
intermarginal space tends to be light gray
marked plastic effect
Polibar ACB
suspended with simple manual shaking
tannic acid is not tolerated
administered by gravity
easily performed colon emptying
no air bubble formation
marked air/barium levels
thin coating
intermarginal space tends to be dark gray
poor plastic effect

pended, like carboxymethylcellulose used in Barotrast. The chain may also be broken before, through special procedures (aquated gums), like in Polibar.

Therefore, for preparation of *Barotrast* suspension intense shaking is required, possibly with a blender. It is thus advisable to prepare the suspension much in advance. It tends to form troublesome air bubbles, for which the addition of an antifoaming agent is required. When used in aqueous suspensions with a concentration ranging from 50 to 65% w/v, it coats the mucosa with thick layers creating intense three-dimensional plastic effects in the X-ray image. Because of the thick coating, the intermarginal space acquires a light-gray background color, hiding the innominate grooves and sometimes also small size polyps. Conversely, the iconographic demonstration of early IUC stages and Crohn's disease is excellent.

The short-chained *Polibar* can be suspended with brief manual shaking; it can thus be prepared on the spot without problems, also because almost no foam is formed. Used in 100% w/v concentration (which means adding 300 mL of water to the 400 g of barium sulfate, to obtain a total volume of 400 mL), it forms 3-4 times thinner coating layers than Barotrast when used at the above mentioned concentrations. The radiographic background color of the intermarginal space is rather dark-gray, thus

making the high kilovoltage radiographic technique particularly useful. In this way also the smallest polyps can be demonstrated. The iconographic demonstration of early IUC stages and Crohn's disease is good.

Generally speaking, the opinion on the results obtained with these two barium suspensions is probably a matter of personal preference for a thicker or thinner layer, for a more or less intense plastic effect, for a poorly spontaneously contrasted image or made so while the X-ray image is being taken [3].

In order to make a more objective evaluation, we have directly compared Barotrast with Polibar in a single-blind experiment on 158 patients to whom the DCBE examination had been specifically prescribed. The double contrast images obtained have been classified according to their quality, meaning, by this term, their higher or lower capacity to yield information useful for the diagnosis. Where possible, purely esthetic elements were neglected. The patients have been randomized, by draw, into two groups for examination with Barotrast (65% w/v suspension) or Polibar (100% w/v suspension). The conventional bowel preparation technique was employed (low-residue diet; castor oil in the afternoon of the day prior to the examination; cleansing enema the evening before and 3 hours before examination). The examination technique was the same as the one described in Chapter 4.

The evaluation of results was done after every examination by two radiologists who did not know which barium suspension had been used. Judgments on the quality of results were then made in accordance with the following scoring :

excellent = uniform mucosal coating, of sufficient thickness to perfectly demonstrate intermarginal spaces, no tendency to mask or cancel any image in the mucosa surface for excessive radiopacity or excessive radiotransparency.

good = coating as above, yet without the three-dimensional "plus" of the image, probably of purely esthetic nature.

fair = some weak points in the barium coating (too thick, or too thin, with evident differences among the various segments of the large intestine) or in excessive air/barium levels which may become troublesome for a correct evaluation of the various colonic segments.

poor = no reliable diagnosis is possible due to the intolerably high degree of above described defects.

No substantial difference was observed between the two barium suspensions ($\chi^2 = 1.058$; P = .90). The most important differential feature emerging from this trial refers to mucosal coating: thick but low density layer with Barotrast; thin but high density layer with Polibar (Fig. 1). The fact that such a difference has no major repercussions on the diagnostic results would reasonably confirm what has already been mentioned above, namely that choosing either of the two suspensions is only a matter of personal preference.

In our experience, however, Polibar offers some advantages over the other product in the type of package: it is supplied in powder form in a single bag which can be used for both suspension preparation as well as enema irrigator for an administration "by gravity" and also, if desired, for the following "closed circuit" drainage of surplus free barium in the colonic lumen. However, with the conventional bowel preparation technique (which, as seen in Chapter 10, is not the one suggested by us), minimum 600 g of barium sulfate should be made available in a single bag in order to obtain at least a 600 mL 100% w/v suspension. With reference to Barotrast, in our opinion, the major disadvantages are the need to use a pressure injector (which is due to the excessive viscosity of the suspension) and its tendency to form foam and air bubbles.

Several opinions of DCBE advocates have pointed out that the mucosal coating obtained with

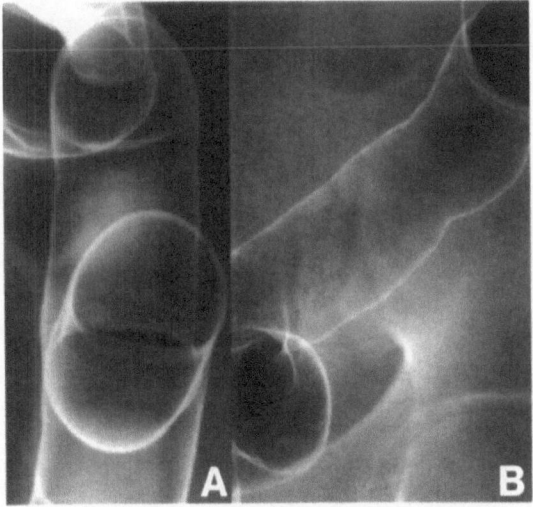

Fig. 1. Typical mucosal coating obtained with Barotrast 65% w/v (**A**) and Polibar ACB 100% w/v (**B**), after conventional bowel preparation (castor oil and cleansing enemas)

Polibar used as described above, may sometimes be too thin. Based on this remark, we have started, by progressive corrective modifications first on the barium formulation, and then on the large bowel cleansing technique (where we have achieved better results), to modify mucosal coating features until the minimum thickening would be achieved, which is required to obtain a good plastic effect in the radiographs.

We started from an easily repeatable experimental observation [4]. By adding 30 g of $MgSO_4$ to 400 ml of 100% w/v Polibar ACB suspension, this tends to rapidly clot into a semisolid paste. Then, with the addition of a proper amount of water, a suitably homogeneous suspension is generally obtained again. Being a reversible phenomenon, we would assume that molecules of free water are being subtracted from the suspending medium by Mg^{++} ions known for their strong hydrophilic properties. The likely interaction between Mg^{++} ions and barium suspensions has been recently suggested also by other Authors [5].

Recently, we evaluated *in vitro* the viscosity of a 80% w/v Polibar ACB suspension, to different samples of which magnesium sulfate, or sodium sulfate as control, was added in quantities increasing from 0.75 to 3.75 g/100 g [6]. Measures were performed also on the supernatant of the suspension after centrifugation. Only a slight increase of viscosity was observed after addition of Na_2SO_4, while after addition of $MgSO_4$ viscosity increased exponentially from the basal value of 50 cPs to 1338 cPs at 20°C, and from 32 to 2398 cPs at 37°C. No substantial effect was observed on the supernatant. No thixotropic effect was observed. The increase of viscosity is evidently due to Mg^{++} ions, since no effect is observed with Na^+ ions at identical concentrations. The effect seems due to water subtraction to the suspending phase, but a complex interaction with the polysaccharidic chain in presence of barium particles cannot be excluded.

We also wanted to verify what would happen in radiological practice by using a more diluted Polibar ACB suspension in patients who had been following the sennosides/$MgSO_4$ bowel preparation protocol described in Chapter 10. As demonstrated by preliminary magnesium assays in the wash-out liquid obtained from the colon at the end of intestinal preparation, a significant amount of residual Mg^{++} ions were indeed found in the colonic lumen [4].

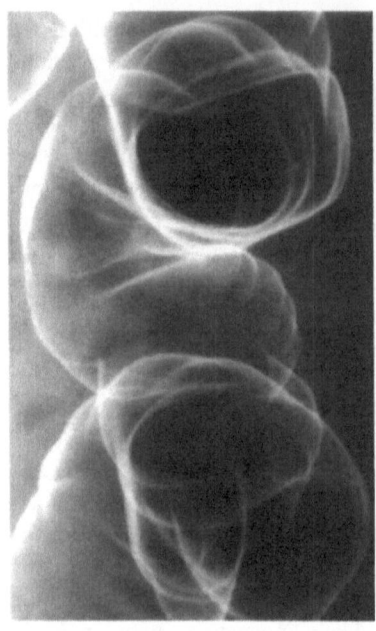

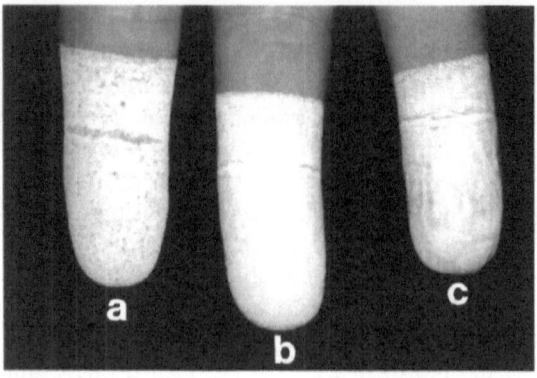

Fig. 3. Adhesiveness to the skin of Polibar ACB 57% w/v (**A**) is somewhat irregular and cribriform, becomes optimal after addition of 15 g $MgSO_4$ to 400 g $BaSO_4$ (**B**), and worsens after addition of 30 g $MgSO_4$ (**C**).

Fig. 2. Typical mucosal coating obtained with Polibar ACB 57% w/v, after bowel preparation according to the Genoa protocol (sennosides and magnesium sulfate)

With the use of a 57% w/v Polibar ACB suspension, the results obtained were particularly encouraging. Since the suspension viscosity is reduced, it moves rapidly and easily along the colon and, after interaction with Mg^{++} ions, it "thickens" *in vivo* with all the benefits of a dense suspension. Probably also due to some changes in the way barium sulfate adheres to the mucosa in the presence of Mg^{++}, the colonic mucosa coating acquires a nice plastic effect (Fig. 2). Variations in adhesiveness are well demonstrated in a simple way when applied to the skin (Fig. 3).

The Genoa technique with the use of Polibar ACB, which is based on the above interpretation, is currently used almost everywhere in Italy: it fully benefits from the advantages obtained with the association between the sennosides/$MgSO_4$ bowel preparation and the use of a more fluid Polibar suspension. A good hydration of the patient is important to ensure that no water is subtracted from the barium suspension by the colonic mucosa. In patients prepared with other associations of cathartics, and, in any case, with cleansing enemas, Polibar ACB will obviously be used with a 100% w/v concentration: in this case, the quality of wall coating will be as described in Table 1 and shown in Fig. 1.

References

1. Cittadini G (1994) Radiologia gastrointestinale - Un crocevia pericoloso: ecoendoscopia o endoecografia? Il Radiologo 33(2):92-94
2. Costanzo C (1979) Associazione Prontobario-Barotrast (lettera). Il Radiologo 18(2):43-44
3. Cittadini G (1979) The blended bariums (answer to 2.). Il Radiologo 18(2):44-45
4. Oliva L, Cittadini G (1981) Il clisma a doppio contrasto: problemi metodologici e tecnici. Verona: Cortina, pp 125-126
5. Conry BG, Jones S, Bartram CI (1981) The effect of oral magnesium-containing bowel preparation agents on mucosal coating by barium sulphate suspensions. Br J Radiol 60:1215-1219
6. Cittadini G, Benatti U, Sardanelli F, De Cicco E (1997) Effects of magnesium on viscosity and thixotropy of barium suspensions. Unpublished data

16 The radiographic recording system

Since the first steps of the Genoa technique, fluoroscopy is used mainly to follow the progress of the barium suspension, and to control the gaseous distention of the colon. It is performed by specifically skilled radiologists or by residents under supervision, but never by radiographers, in spite of the fact that formal training may enable this form of role extension, the radiographer-performed barium enema [1]. From a diagnostic point of view, the evaluation of standard overhead radiographs, each of them supposed to display the whole colon, and, when obtained, of spot radiographs, is of paramount importance. Therefore, particular attention was paid to the radiographic recording system with reference to contrast, resolution and format.

In Chapter 4, the choice of a high kilovoltage radiographic technique was mentioned. The selection of this element is somehow interconnected to that of rare earth screens required for the best technical use of high radiographic voltages (120 kVp), without having to resort to grids with a too high ratio. With high kilovoltage radiography, the image contrast, which is generally high in DCBE, can be reduced. Anyway, the features required for the image recording system in DCBE deserve a more detailed examination.

The screen/film system is an integral element of the whole radiographic system which affects the quality of final images significantly. It works as a *receiver*, by collecting the X-ray beam which is being modulated by its passage through the body area under investigation, as *transformer*, by transforming the X-ray energy into light energy, and as *recorder*, by making the radiographic image permanently visible to the radiologist.

The most useful operating conditions to obtain a good quality of the double-contrast images of the colon are: the use of a fine focal spot (0.6 x 0.6 mm); a source-image receptor distance (SID) of 1.2-1.5 m; maximum 0.1 s exposure time; adequate contrast of the final image. Excessively gray and confused images as well as images where the difference between dark and light areas is too striking, should be avoided. In particular, the image must be sufficiently sharp to allow the identification of small details with diagnostic value (fine erosions, 2-3 mm polyps, etc.). At the same time, any intrinsic movement of the parts under examination which, despite the use of appropriate hypokinetic drugs, may still be present during radiological examination, must be kept under control. Also, while taking into account the exposed body volume and the number of radiographs required, the X-ray energy absorbed by the patient must be limited as much as possible (see Chapter 17).

In order to meet all these requirements, an accurate selection of the radiographic recording system is essential, so that a trade-off can be found between the information gathered and its "cost". The above mentioned purpose was the starting point of many research works we performed in collaboration with Imation Italy, at that time 3M Italy.

The intensifying screens consist of three layers placed over a polyester support: an external layer for protection; an intermediate layer, the most important one, containing the phosphor material which, when hit by X-rays, emits light; and finally, an internal layer which reflects the emitted light and prevents its scattering through the support.

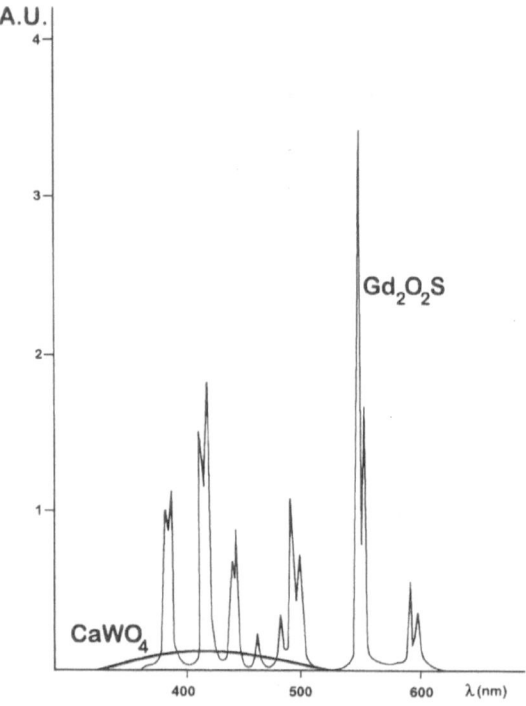

Fig. 1. Emission spectrum of Gd_2O_2S and $CaWO_4$

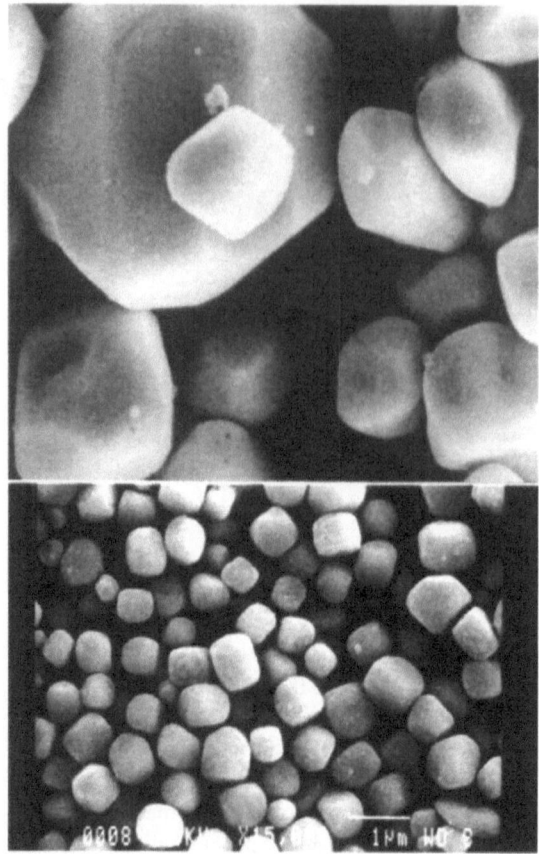

Fig. 2. Size of $CaWO_4$ (top) and Gd_2O_2S (bottom) phosphor crystals. 15.000x magnification

The first difference between *gadolinium oxysulfide* (Gd_2O_2S), the most popular phosphor used in rare earth screens, and *calcium tungstate*, employed in conventional screens, is the wavelength of emitted light: Gd_2O_2S mainly emits in the green, $CaWO_4$ in the blue (Fig. 1).

As a consequence of the wavelength of the light emitted by Gd_2O_2S, a corresponding sensitization is required for the films to be used in association with it. The second difference is the size of phosphor crystals: Gd_2O_2S crystals are smaller and more regular than $CaWO_4$ ones, thus finding easier arrangement in the fluorescent layer (Fig. 2).

However, the fundamental difference between the two types of screens, the one that has mostly contributed to the successful propagation of rare earth screens over conventional ones, is their difference phosphor performance, which is expressed as the product of three factors: ability to absorb X-rays (absorption), ability to transform X-rays into light (conversion), and ability to transmit emitted light (transmission):

$$E = A \times C \times T$$

Since absorption and especially conversion are higher in Gd_2O_2S than $CaWO_4$, while transmission is almost the same, Gd_2O_2S performance is greater than $CaWO_4$. In concrete terms, a Gd_2O_2S rare earth screen can return back as light 7% of the energy received in the form of X-rays, vs. 1.1% of a conventional $CaWO_4$ screen with the same structure [2].

Obviously enough, the greater efficiency of rare earth phosphors vs. conventional can be used either to produce screens with higher light emission for an equal amount of incident X-rays, or to produce screens which, though thinner, emit the same amount of light. In the first case, exposure is reduced with subsequent reduction in the amount of X-ray energy absorbed by the patient, without any loss of image quality; in the second case, image quality is improved without changing the exposure dose.

In our opinion and as better illustrated in Chapter 17 in the case of DCBE examination, exposure reduction is first and foremost to be preferred. By using 600-speed rare earth radiographic systems, radiographs can be obtained requiring 6 times less exposure dose than with a 100-speed conventional system, without any significant reduction in quality. Should a limited loss of quality be acceptable, such exposure can be further reduced, in terms of mAs, though this may perhaps be recommended only in children.

Therefore, in practice, it is possible to reduce the X-ray tube load, so as to be able to use a sufficiently fine spot, together with a short exposure time, so as to decrease the blurring caused by movements, the so called kinetic blurring. At the same time, the possibility to increase the SID will permit to further reduce geometric blurring. Therefore, a proper high speed rare earth system does not only mean reducing the radiation dose to the patient, but also, in the case of DCBE, improving image quality through a better operation control during exposure. As already mentioned, the greatest advantage of rare earth systems is perhaps the simplified use, with better results, of the high kilovoltage technique. This is due to their intrinsic filtration effect on scattered radiation of lower energy [3], thus requiring no higher ratio grids (Fig. 3).

Our experience is based on an extensive testing of the most commonly used rare earth systems, and particularly Imation Trimax, Kodak Lanex, and more recently Sterling UltraVision systems.

Imation Trimax proved to be a very flexible and particularly suitable system for the protocol applied in our Genoa technique: i.e., 7 standard radiographs and, when necessary, conventional spot films with medium definition, for which Regular screens (T16 in Italy, T12 in the United States) and XDA Plus APS film are recommended (600-speed system); detail and high definition spot films may be required for individual patients, for which Fine screens (T2) and XDA Plus APS or GTU films are recommended (100-speed or 75-speed system, respectively). The sequence of standard radiographs is developed as soon as possible, to enable the radiologist to immediately decide whether other detail

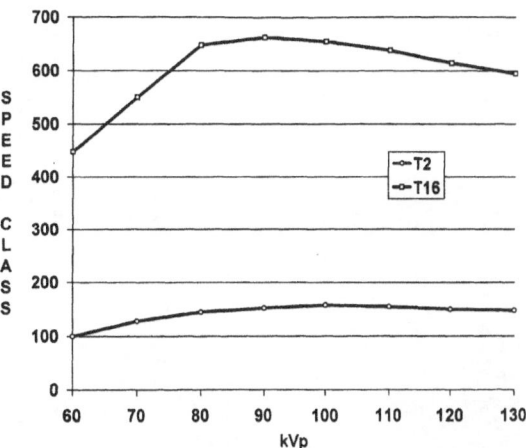

Fig. 3. Intrinsic grid effect of Gd_2O_2S intensifying screens. The Imation Regular (T16) screen sensitivity is significantly reduced in case of an X-ray beam with maximum energy below 80 keV, thus "deleting" some of the scattered radiation. This effect is less evident with Fine (T2) screens

radiographs or spot films are required: a day-light unit for film treatment is undoubtedly useful in this case.

For the high resolution offered by the GTU film, especially confirmed in studies of primary bone structures, we decided to test it extensively in our DCBE examinations, as soon as it was made available on the market. Some examples of the results which can be obtained with T16/XDA and T2/GTU systems are illustrated in Figs. 4 and 5. Despite obvious differences in the quality of images being compared, our practical experience has confirmed that these differences are unlikely to affect diagnostic information. In other words, images that are "far too beautiful" may be easy on the eye of the radiologist, but fail to give any additional information on small polyps, on the progression of IUC front, or when examining peculiar findings like the innominate grooves, submucosal lymphoid hyperplasia, relief alterations of mucosal folds.

The Kodak Lanex system is used with Regular screens and TMAT/G film (400-speed), or Fine screens and TMAT/G film (100-speed). The Sterling UltraVision system is used with U-V Rapid screens and UVG film (400-speed).

The use of wide latitude films, such as Imation XLA Plus APS, Kodak TMAT/L and Sterling UVL has also yielded interesting results [4]. Having a less steep contrast slope, minor exposure defects can

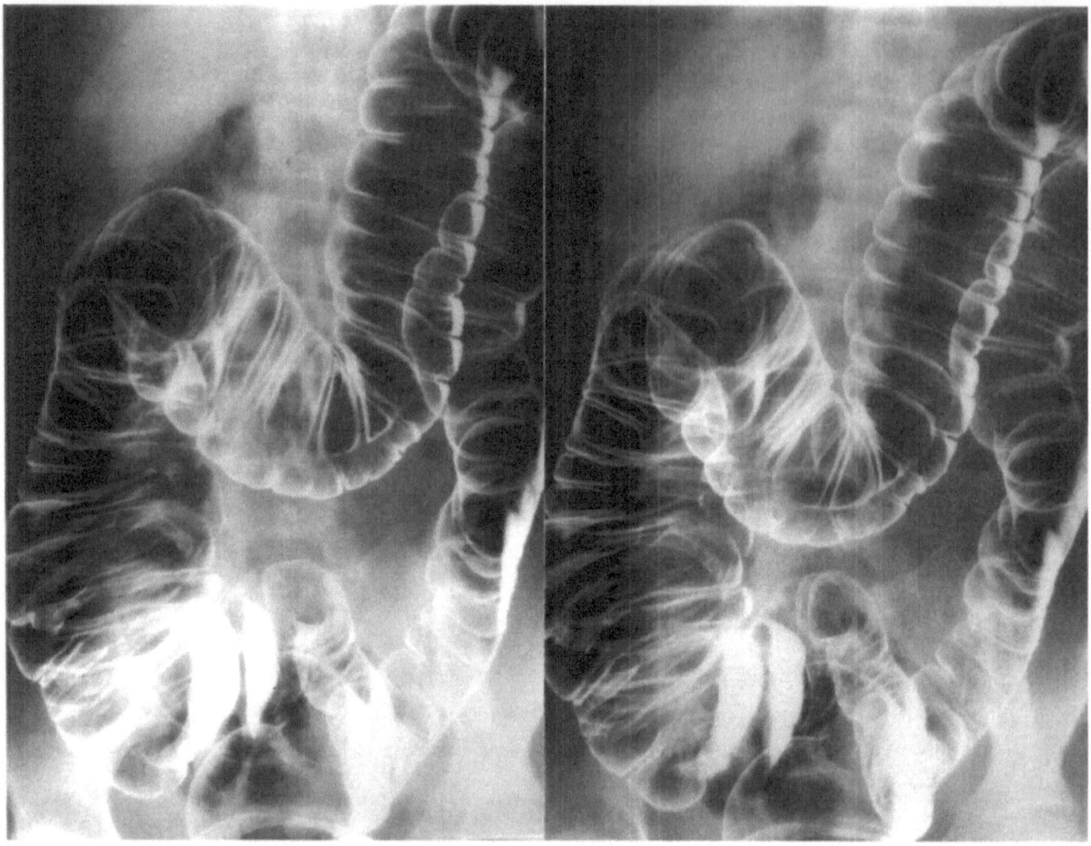

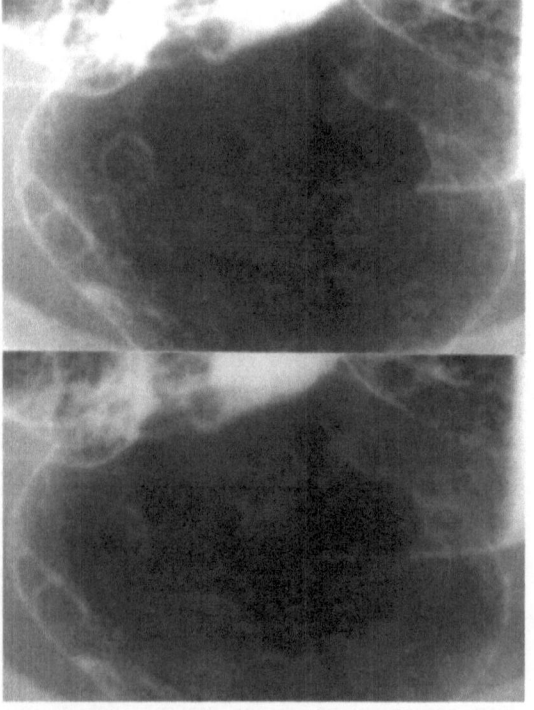

Fig. 4. Image quality when using medium definition Imation T16+XDA Plus APS (*left*) and high definition T2+GTU (*right*) rare earth systems. Both images have a high quality level and no additional information is given by the higher definition image. X-ray exposure: 120 kVp and 4 mAs (*left*); 120 kVp and 32 mAs (*right*)

Fig. 5. Familial adenomatous polyposis. Detail of the rectum. *Top*: radiograph as in Fig. 4 left; *bottom*: radiograph as in Fig. 4 right

better be offset, whereas with standard latitude films additional radiographs would have to be taken.

The need to obtain spot radiographs is often due to the fact that the whole colon cannot be fully displayed in the 14" x 17" format. Practical experience demonstrates that the distance from the lowest point of the large bowel (the anal canal) and the highest (the left flexure) is often greater than the maximal lenght of conventional radiographic formats (17"). In a recent survey [5], the large bowel was fully displayed (from the rectum to the left flexure) in 21.6% of supine antero-posterior, 24.3% of prone postero-anterior, and 35.1% of upright postero-anterior radiographic images. One segment (rectum or left flexure) was cut in 51.4%, 45.9% and 43.3%, respectively; both rectum and left flexure were cut in 27.0%, 29.8% and 21.6%, respectively.

We have evaluated a new radiographic format consisting of a 16" x 20" cassette containing a Imation rare earth 600-speed screen/film system optimized for 120 KVp X-ray photons. Owing to the impossibility to expose the film in the usual way (Potter-Bucky grid; cassette into the radiographic table), an intracassette 16" x 20" fixed grid in carbon fiber of special design (12:1 ratio; focus at 180 cm, valid range 138-257 cm), obtained by Gilardoni (Mandello Lario, Italy), was used. The cassette was placed directly under the patient's body surface. Images obtained with the larger format were quite similar to those obtained with the conventional format for what concerns contrast and sharpness. The large bowel was nearly always displayed from top to bottom [5], increasing the number of complete images of the rectum and left flexure in the radiographic sequence. How important this may be to increase the number of pathologies discovered is at the moment object of work in progress.

In the Genoa technique no equalizing filters are used for decubitus radiographs [6]. Videotape recording is occasional, cineradiography very rare. Digital fluoroscopic and radiographic systems offer satisfactory results [7-9] but have limitations in the image format [10]. However, their use is becoming more frequent especially for the lower amount of radiation to the patient [7,11-13].

References

1. Bewell J, Chapman AH (1996) Radiographer-performed barium enemas - Results of a survey to assess progress. Radiography 2:199-205
2. Oggioni R (1979) Gli schermi alle terre rare. Radiol Med 65 (Suppl 2):189-193
3. Castle JW (1977) Sensitivity of radiographic screens to scattered radiation and its relationship to image contrast. Radiology 122:805-809
4. Rollandi GA, Gambaro A, Pulzato P et al (1984) Utilizzazione di una pellicola a basso gradiente di contrasto nelle indagini a doppio contrasto del tubo digerente. Radiol Med 70(Suppl 4):89-91
5. Cittadini G, Sardanelli F, De Cicco E et al (1998) A larger film format (16x20 inches) in double-contrast barium enema examination. Br J Radiol (in press)
6. Olson DL, Dodds WJ, Stewart ET et al (1987) Efficacy of an intracassette filter for improved pneumocolon decubitus radiographs. AJR 148:547-549
7. Perri G, Palla L, Battolla L et al (1991) Clisma a doppio contrasto - Studio del disegno mucoso e del profilo d'organo con le metodiche tradizionale e digitale. Radiol Med 81:844-848
8. Okada Y, Kusano S, Endo T (1994) Double-contrast barium enema study with computed radiography: assessment in detection of colorectal polyps. J Digit Imaging 7:154-159
9. Barkhof F, David E, De Geest F (1996) Comparison of film-screen combination and digital fluorography in gastrointestinal barium examinations in a clinical setting. Eur J Radiol; 22:232-235
10. Bellomi M, Severini A, Cozzi G et al (1994) La fluoroscopia digitale nella radiologia gastroenterologica. Radiol Med 87:460-468
11. Kastan DJ, Ackerman LV, Feczko PJ (1987) Digital gastrointestinal imaging: The effect of pixel size on detection of subtle mucosal abnormalities. Radiology 162:853-856
12. Krug B, Steinbrich W, Lorenz R et al (1990) Kolonkontrasteinlauf in digitaler lumineszenradiographie (DLR) und konventioneller röntgentechnik. Fortschr Geb Rontgenstr Nuklearmed; 152:131-136
13. Zonca G, Brusa A, Bellomi M et al (1995) Absorbed dose to the skin in radiological examinations of upper and lower gastrointestinal tract. Radiat Prot Dosim 57:489-492

17 DCBE and risk of radioinduced somatic and genetic damage

Giampiero Tosi

In daily clinical practice, dosimetric aspects of roentgenologic examinations are often neglected. Also in radiology publications this topic is not discussed so much as it should, except for some general remarks referring to the various types of examinations as a whole. Perhaps this attitude is due to the fact that the radiologist has become somehow familiar with an invisible enemy, whose action is difficult to relate to immediate damage.

On the one side, the radiologist, focused on the solution of diagnostic problems, is likely to overdo the iconography acquisition, either out of zeal or out of an esthetic search [1,2], thus forgetting that what he is doing is not without risks. On the other hand, however, an unclear knowledge of the real risks involved in a roentgenologic examination may lead physicians as well as patients to fear ionizing radiations in a really superstitious way, thus hampering an objective trade-off between diagnostic benefits and acceptable risks involved.

All modern methods for roentgenologic investigations of the digestive tract involve a fluoroscopic and a radiographic phase. DCBE is not exempted from this rule: therefore, the accurate dosimetry of both components is essential.

Generally speaking, the values indicated in the literature mainly refer to the *surface dose* (Fig. 1), namely the radiation dose received by the patient's body surface from the incident beam and through back-scattering from underlying tissues. However, the surface dose parameter fails to consider the depth transmission of X-rays [3], the size of the irradiated field as well as other important factors required to determine the total amount of energy released from the radiation beam.

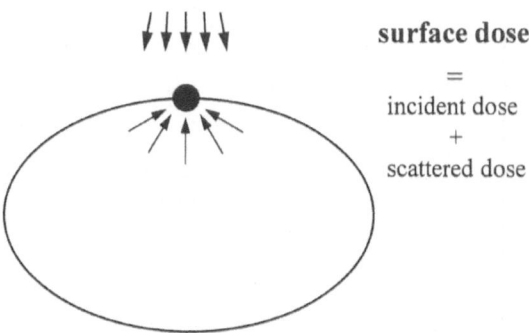

Fig. 1. Surface dose (see text)

Therefore, when trying to assess the actual risk of radiation damage, the *surface dose* alone is not enough, and the *integral dose* must be determined, that is to say the total energy absorbed by the irradiated area (Fig. 2).

Though in risk assessment a linear dose-effect relation is generally applied in a conservative ap-

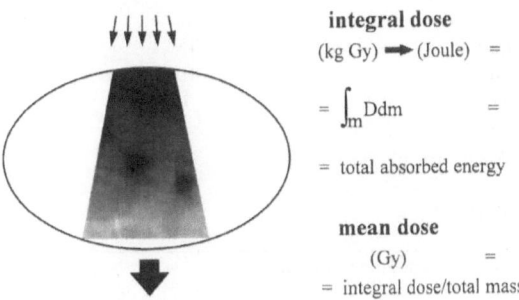

Fig. 2. Integral and mean doses (see text)

proach, a sigma-shaped curve would better represent reality [4] (Fig. 3). Indeed, this curve would correspond, with obvious biological meaning, to a slow risk increase at lower doses, a rapid increase for intermediate doses, a limited additional increase for higher doses, no matter how much the dose is then being raised.

The risk can be conveniently normalized as risk per Gy absorbed by the body or in the target tissue [5]. In Table 1, taken from the issue No. 60 of

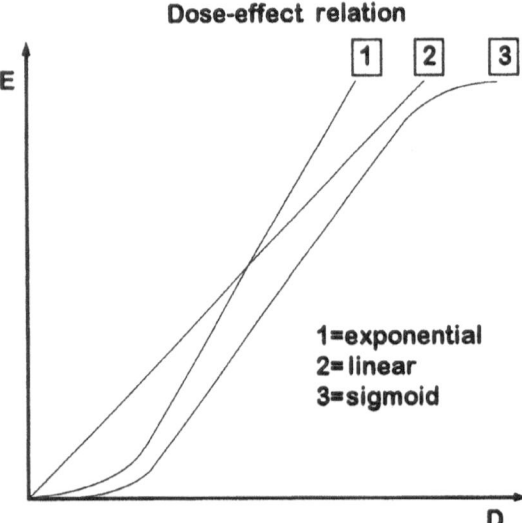

Fig. 3. Possible correlations between X-ray dose and biological effect

ICRP [6], the figures corresponding to the probability of fatal cancer after exposure to low doses of radiation are reported and the relative contribution of various organs to the total detriment. The onset of non lethal tumors and likely severe radioinduced genetic effects have also been considered. From the values indicated, the probability of lethal tumors (for 10^4 people/Sv) is 500: this means that in a population of 10,000 people who have uniformly absorbed 1 Gy of radiation all over their body, there will be 500 more cases of lethal tumors than the background risk. However, it will not be possible to correlate the onset of the disease with past radiation exposure in the individual case, since this type of pathology occurs, in an apparently spontaneous way, also in non exposed individuals. Therefore, only the increase in the incidence of the various tumors depending on this exposure can be calculated.

The figures concerning DCBE are based on calculations which consider radiographic parameters and fluoroscopy doses normally employed in our department, with perfectly calibrated radiation source, rare earth intensifying Trimax Regular screens and XDA Plus APS film. Doses have been calculated for an individual of 65 Kg weight, 20 and 30 cm antero-posterior and latero-lateral body thickness, respectively. The X-ray beam is supposed to be filtered with 2.5 mm Al.

As reported in Table 2 Chapter 4, 7 standard radiographs are required by the Genoa technique. 120 kVp are normally used with an average expo-

Table 1. Probability of fatal cancer after exposure to low doses of radiation and relative contribution of different organs to the total detriment. (From *ICRP publication No. 60*)

Organ	Probability of fatal cancer (per 10^4 people/Sv)	Severe genetic effects (per 10^4 people/Sv)	Relative contribution
Bladder	30		0.040
Bone marrow	50		0.143
Bone surface	5		0.009
Colon	85		0.141
Liver	15		0.122
Ovary[1]	10		0.020
Skin	2		0.006
Gonads[1]		100	0.183
Remainder	303		0.336
Total	500		1.000

[1] Gonads (including cancer in ovary)

sure of 4 mAs in sagittal projections (No. 1, 2, 4, 5 and 6), 14 mAs in semiaxial projections (No. 3), and 18 mAs in latero-lateral projections of the rectosigmoid junction (No. 7). Spot films and additional radiographs have not been considered, though their contribution to the total dose is undoubtedly significant, especially when they are obtained with less rapid recording systems in order to improve the definition. SID is 120 cm. A tipping table with a 12:1 ratio Potter-Bucky grid is always employed.

As illustrated in Table 2, where all intermediate calculations have also been indicated, the mean total dose for the radiographic component alone amounts to 2.56 mGy, which is low, yet not very low. Conversely, the dose deriving from fluoroscopy is much higher: in DCBE it may be 50% higher than in SCBE when the intensifier aperture and TV tube ratio is not properly set. With the same filtration as mentioned above, with a 24 x 30 cm field size, 100 kVp and 1 mA, the surface dose amounts to 14.85 mGy each minute of fluoroscopy; the mean dose is therefore 2.2 mGy/mA/minute.

Actually, the majority of equipments with a brilliance intensifier is also equipped with a control system enhancing, at equal voltage, the current intensity to the tube which, on average, reaches 1.8 mA. Hence, with these parameters, the mean dose amounts to 4 mGy. Therefore, in one minute of fluoroscopy, the mean dose is about 1.5 times the total radiographic dose. Hence, the need to reduce fluoroscopy time rather than the number of radiographs. Just imagine that it takes from 2 to 3 minutes of fluoroscopy for all the controls required during the double contrast implementation phase.

If, for the standard radiographic sequence, conventional screens or low rather than high speed rare earth intensifier screens are used, the dose amount deriving from radiography is 6 times higher [7]. In other words, this would be equal to 4-5 more minutes of fluoroscopy.

When calculating the leukemogenesis risk (Table 3) it must be kept in mind that, in the adult, the pelvis contains 50% of active hematopoietic marrow. Since the average dose on the marrow is 24 mGy, the leukemogenic risk, or total leukemia induction probability, can be calculated as follows: out of 10,000 individuals undergoing DCBE with the above described technical features, 1 more case of leukemia can occur within 5-10 years since exposure. The bone carcinogenesis risk is of 1 more tumor case in 1 million exposed people, with 20 year risk duration. The global radiological risk is obviously higher: out of 10,000 individuals exposed to DCBE, there will be 5 more tumor cases for the entire life duration.

Finally, the risk of genetic damage within the second generation is about 4×10^{-4}. The incidence

Table 2. DCBE - Genoa technique - Dose to the patient

A) **Radiography** (total filtration = 2.5 mm Al; Imation Trimax Regular + XDA Plus APS)

Standard radiographs	kV	mAs	SSD	Exp. (mR)	Rxcm²	f_i	ID (Kg - Gy)	Mean dose (µGy)
1, 2, 4, 5, 6	120	4	100	170	0.170x1050	8.6	1.535×10^{-2}	236
3	120	14	100	580	0.580x1050	9.0	5.481×10^{-2}	843
7	120	18	90	900	0.900x 405	9.5	3.463×10^{-2}	533

Total mean dose = (236x5) + (843x1) + (533x1) µGy = 2.56 mGy

B) **Fluoroscopy** (total filtration = 2.5 mm Al; field of view 24 x 30 cm)

kV	Surface dose (mGy/mA x min)	Mean dose (mGy/mA x min)
100	14.85	2.20

1 min fluoroscopy with 1.8 mA = Mean dose = 4 mGy
Total mean dose = 4 mGy x 3 min = 12 mGy

SSD = source - skin distance; f_i = integral dose factor; ID = integral dose

Table 3. DCBE - Genoa technique - Doses and risks

Actually irradiated mass = 20 kg
Total local mean dose = 8.32 mGy (radiography) + 39 mGy (3' fluoroscopy) = 47.32 mGy
Irradiated fraction of active bone marrow = 50%
Marrow mean dose = 47.32 mGy x 0.5 = 23.66 mGy
Leukemogenic risk = 10^{-4}
Bone cancer risk = 10^{-6}
Global radiologic risk (radiography + 3' fluoroscopy) = 5×10^{-4}

in females is likely to be higher, since gonads cannot be shielded. Therefore the use of postero-anterior projections is recommended in women as much as possible, resulting in approximately a two thirds radiation reduction to the ovaries, being protected by the pelvis bones. Though the dose to hematopoietic marrow is thus increased, the greater leukemogenesis risk of this solution is offset by a reduction in the genetic risk in fertile age women.

If high speed radiographic recording systems are not used, or when radiography or fluoroscopy is excessively used, or even when the equipment employed has no brilliance intensifier, all the above mentioned risk values are likely to increase even by one order of magnitude. The use of digital radiographic systems seems to offer some opportunity to reduce the radiation dose [8].

On the whole, apart from useless alarmist attitudes, DCBE can be rightly considered as an examination which, from the point of view of radio-induced damage risks, can be carried out with a good level of confidence, provided the above recommended technical measures are scrupulously followed [9].

References

1. Eisenberg RL, Hedgcock MW (1981) Preliminary radiograph for barium enema examination: Is it necessary? AJR 136:115-116
2. Eisenberg RL, Meyers PC, May ST (1983) Optimum overhead views in double-contrast barium-enema examinations. AJR 140:595-606
3. Bednarek DR, Rudin S, Wong R (1983) Assessment of patient exposure for barium enema examination. Invest Radiol 18:453-458
4. Wachsmann F, Drexler G (1976) Graphs and tables for use in radiology. Berlin: Springer, pp 57-59
5. Gregg EC (1977) Radiation risks with diagnostic x-rays. Radiology 123:447-453
6. ICRP publication 60 (1990) Annals of the ICRP. Oxford: Pergamon Press, p 136
7. Tosi G (1979) Le terre rare: considerazioni protezionistiche. Radiol Med 65(Suppl 2):193-198
8. Krug B, Steinbrich W, Lorenz R et al (1990) Kolonkontrasteinlauf in digitaler Lumineszenradiographie (DLR) und konventioneller Röntgentechnik. Fortschr Geb Rontgenstr Nuklearmed 152:131-136
9. Cittadini G, Garlaschi G, Sartoris F (1979) Le terre rare: approccio biologico. Radiol Med 65(Suppl 2):198-201

18 Barium enema examination of the colon in children

Children are not adults in miniature, but developing organisms: hence, in pediatrics, radiological studies of any organ generally have to face rapidly changing normal conditions [1]. The peculiar behaviors of pediatric patients, the need for special adjustments in methodology and technique, the unique and constantly changing assessment parameters between normal and pathologic conditions (for example, in the pediatric colon, an apparently lymphoid hyperplasia could well be a normal follicular pattern, even when accompanied by rectal bleeding [2-4]), the peculiar features of many pathologic forms (and congenital malformations in particular), all require a highly specialized approach in the study of the colon.

Although virtually all diseases concerning the colon and rectum in the adults may affect children as well [5], the DCBE is to be prescribed only in carefully selected situations [6-8]. The type of examination (instant enema, SCBE, DCBE) and the need, if any, of bowel preparation [9] will be determined and based upon the age of the patient, on a preliminary clinical picture with an accurate diagnostic frame and on the findings of the plain film of chest-abdomen.

The *plain film of chest-abdomen*, while absolutely fundamental in the case of acute abdomen, becomes important in Chilaiditi's syndrome, in suspected IUC, Crohn's disease and necrotizing enterocolitis. Important information can also be acquired in constipation cases on the amount and distribution of intestinal residues, on the presence of subocclusions, or associated vertebral malformations.

The *therapeutic enema*, performed with water-soluble iodinated contrast medium, is used in ileo-colonic intussusception, in meconium ileum, and milk and meconium plug syndromes.

Generally, SCBE without any particular bowel preparation is the method of choice in infants in the assessment of morphologic variations of the colon, stenoses, constipation, Hirschsprung's disease (where laxatives and cleansing enemas are contraindicated since they can decompress the colon above the aganglionic segment, thus hindering any correct definition of the transition area), in post-surgery controls. DCBE, since requires a rigorous preparation like in the adult patient, is the method of choice in children from 3-4 years old, and is employed to study inflammatory diseases (Fig. 1), polyps and tumors (Fig. 2) and in late follow-up of anastomoses. The higher sensitivity of DCBE over SCBE has been demonstrated in early IUC stages and Crohn's disease [10]. The good correlation between DCBE and colonoscopy reports confirms the validity of DCBE in pediatric patients [11-13].

When planning a DCBE examination, bowel preparation is the most delicate phase, being generally more difficult than in the adult, mainly because of a low compliance of the young patient and his/her parents. The possibility of obtaining good results in pediatric patients by using purely pharmacological bowel preparation protocols without cleansing enemas was reported by some Authors [14]. The Genoa technique [15] with proper modifications to posology (Table 1), is routinely used at the Giannina Gaslini Children Hospital of Genoa, and it has helped to obtain a clean colon in 90% of cases. In the remaining 10%, a proper evaluation is usually not hindered by fecal residues. No significant side effects have been reported.

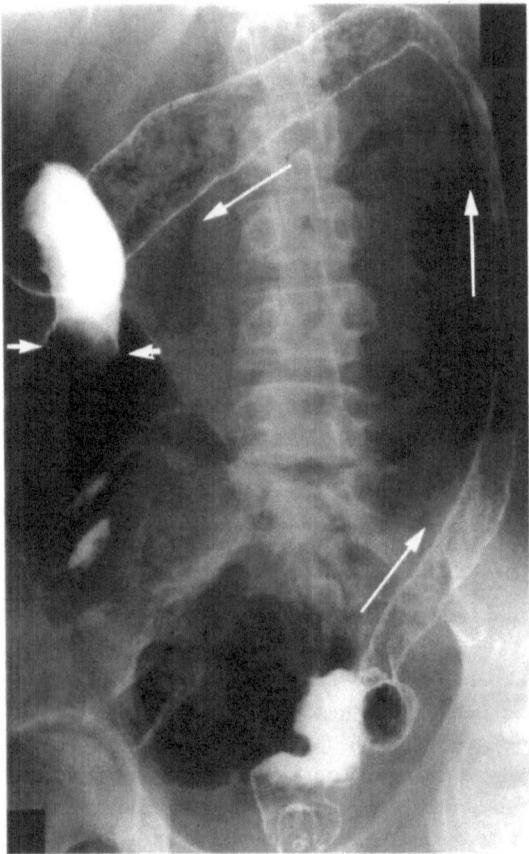

Fig. 1. IUC in 12 years old child. The disease progress (*long arrows*) stops at the level of the upper portion of the ascending colon (*short arrows*). The portion beneath, though significantly dilated, is unaffected

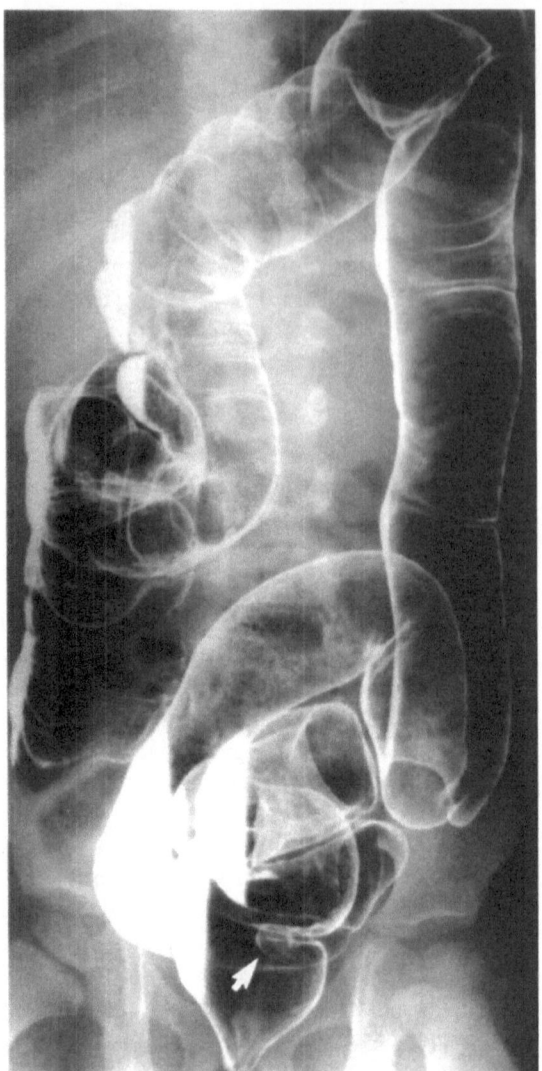

Fig. 2. With a good bowel preparation and the overall view of the large bowel, it was possible to detect a single pedunculated polyp (*arrow*) located in the lower portion of the rectal ampulla

The conventional protocol featuring castor oil (1-5 mL per day in sucklings and 5-15 mL in weaned children) and a cleansing enema (lukewarm physiological saline solution at least 5 hours before the radiological examination), is day by day becoming obsolete in Italy.

A good colon hypotony is recommended in children too. We prefer to use atropine sulfate *per os*, at a reduced dose according to Welin's suggestion [16]: 0.25 mg in children 3 to 6 years old; 0.50 mg in children 6 to 9 years old; 0.75 mg in children 9 to 12 years old; 1 mg in children older than 12 years.

If i.m. administration is preferred, 0.01 mg/Kg body weight are administered. Hyoscine N-butylbromide (Buscopan) is a good alternative to at-

ropine, given i.v. (0.2 mg/Kg body weight) immediately before gaseous insufflation of the colon.

During the examination, particular attention will be paid to the issue of radiation protection[17]. The anti-scatter grid should be avoided; proper shielding is required all around the organ to be investigated during radiography and fluoroscopy; the duration of fluoroscopy should be reduced as much as possible as well as the number of radiographs. High speed screen/film systems are always recommended.

Table 1. Bowel preparation protocol in children according to the Genoa technique

During the 3 days preceding the examination: low-residue diet

1 day before:

8	a.m.	X-Prep 1 mL/Kg of body weight
12	a.m.	diet as above
5	p.m.	$MgSO_4$ 0.20 g/Kg of body weight
5-8	p.m.	hydration (1 liter of water)

Fast until examination
No cleansing enema

We use the same radiographic sequence employed in the adult, as described in Chapter 4. In the lateral projection of the recto-sigmoid with horizontal beam, the elevation of the buttocks (knee-chest view) allows barium to drain retrogradely from the air-filled rectum, improving its visualization in selected patients [18].

References

1. de Filippi G (1995) Radiologia pediatrica. In: Cittadini G Manuale di Diagnostica per immagini e radioterapia. Genova: Ecig, p 721

2. Capitanio MA, Kirkpatrick JA (1970) Lymphoid hyperplasia of the colon in children. Radiology 94:323-327

3. Laufer I, deSa D (1978) Lymphoid follicular pattern: A normal feature of the pediatric colon. AJR 130:51-55

4. Riddlesberger MM Jr, Lebenthal E (1980) Nodular colonic mucosa of childhood: normal or pathologic? Gastroenterology 79:265-270

5. Singleton EB, Johnson F (1976) Localized lesions of the colon in infants and children. Semin Roentgenol 11(2):162-170

6. Astley R (1975) Radiology of intestinal tract. In: Anderson C and Burke V, Pediatric Gastroenterology. Oxford: Blackwell

7. Singleton EB, Wagner ML, Dutton RV (1977) Radiology of the alimentary tract in infants and children. Philadelphia: Saunders,

8. Franken EA Jr, Smith WL (1982) Gastrointestinal imaging in pediatrics. Philadelphia: Harper&Row Publ

9. Tamburrini O, Del Vecchio E, Sodano A (1983) Clisma in età pediatrica: tecnica e metodica. Napoli: Idelson

10. Winthrop JD, Balfe DM, Shackelford GD et al (1985) Ulcerative and granulomatous colitis in children - Comparison of double- and single-contrast studies. Radiology 154:657-660

11. Gugliantini P, Barbuti D, Bergami GL (1982) Radiologia vs endoscopia nella diagnostica dell'apparato digerente: il punto di vista del radiologo. Rass It Chir Ped 24(Suppl 4):11-16

12. Stringer DA, Sherman PM, Jakowenko N (1986) Correlation of double-contrast high-density barium enema, colonoscopy, and histology in children with special attention to disparities. Pediatr Radiol 16:298-301

13. Aggarwal V, Mitta SK, Kumar N et al (1995) A comparative study of double contrast barium enema and colonoscopy for evaluation of rectal bleeding in children. Trop Gastroenterol 16:132-137

14. Reither M (1980) Experiences with Cascara-Salax® preparating children for barium enema (Germ). Rontgenbl 33:418-421

15. Cittadini G, Rollandi GA, Giribaldi M (1980) Su un metodo semplice, innocuo ed efficiente di pulizia intestinale senza clisteri. Radiol Med 66:415-420

16. Welin S, Welin G (1976) The double-contrast examination of the colon. Experience with the Welin modification. Stuttgart: Thieme

17. de Filippi G, Gallo E, Gugliantini P et al (1986) Radiologia pediatrica - Apparato digerente: Standards metodologici. Napoli: Idelson

18. Bowen A III (1979) Double-contrast enemas in children: the "knee-chest" view of the rectosigmoid colon. Pediatr Radiol 8:225-226

19 DCBE and irritable bowel syndrome: only negative signs?

The irritable bowel syndrome (IBS) is a functional intestinal disorder with chronic or recurrent gastrointestinal symptoms without structural or biochemical abnormalities [1]. Abdominal pain is the prominent feature, associated with diarrhea, or constipation, or both; painless diarrhea and simple constipation are excluded from IBS. Gut dysmotility in IBS is affected by stimuli such as food, hormones, drugs, menses, mechanical distention, psychological stress.

Symptoms consistent with a diagnosis of IBS are present in almost one quarter of the population and tend to be associated with a number of other complaints and conditions outside the intestine, some of which may reflect smooth muscle dysfunction [2]. From 30% to 70% of all outpatients consulting a gastroenterologist turn out to be affected by IBS [3-5]. The social importance of this syndrome is great, since IBS in some countries is the second cause of absenteeism from work [3,6].

A positive clinical diagnosis is generally feasible, according to Manning's criteria [7], thus reducing the amount of investigation in many patients with chronic abdominal pain. However, preliminarily, it is always necessary to exclude organic diseases of the colon and organs such as the gallbladder, biliary tree, duodenum, pancreas, uterus and adnexa, which may induce reflex colonic symptoms.

Traditionally, radiology has been applied to rule out the presence of organic diseases, thus having an *indirect* diagnostic role. Conversely, its ability to display *direct* signs of abnormal colonic motility is not much appreciated, mainly because, in the past, some radiological changes observed at barium ex-

aminations were attributed to the use of cathartics and enemas, to the temperature of the barium suspension and to aggressive palpation of the colon during fluoroscopy [4].

Anyway, the presence of luminal narrowing, increased number of haustra and segmental spasm are considered to be a strong radiological evidence of the IBS, provided that the barium enema is performed with a single-contrast technique and any strong bowel preparation is avoided [8]. The segmental areas of spasm particularly affect the sigmoid colon [5]. Rapid filling, areas of irritability and spasm, and increased segmentation become significant if the patient experiences distress coupled to clinical complaints [9]. Sigmoid contractions coupled with pain have been observed in some cases of irritable bowel syndrome [10]. Prediverticulosis may follow a long lasting clinical pattern of IBS [8,11].

According to Kelvin and Gardiner [12], the SCBE approach involves an unacceptable risk of missing underlying organic lesions: a DCBE examination should be performed, instead, using a thorough bowel preparation.

The whole issue can be examined from a different point of view. The double-contrast study directly displays structures related to colonic motility such as haustral pouches, semilunar folds, pseudosphincters, pseudoplicar formations of the mucosa. Therefore, changes in these structures should be easily and more frequently detectable in patients whose final diagnosis is IBS.

On this subject, previous reports [13,14] drew the attention to some motoric patterns of the colon, such as diffuse spasm or distention (Fig. 1), local hypersegmentation (Fig. 2), persistent narrowed annular segments which can simulate organic disease of the colon [15-17] (Fig. 3), pseudoplicar formations of the mucosa looking like multiple intersecting loops or with a clear coil-shaped pattern (Fig. 4).

A special importance was attached to pseudoplicar formations, mainly for their elevated frequency. These formations, sometimes localized and just appreciable (Fig. 5), sometimes very showy (Fig. 6; see also Fig. 3 in Chapter 3), may fail to induce any caliber reduction of the segment concerned, or contour alterations, or haustral segmentation. They can be easily differentiated from semilunar folds by the absence of any rail track pattern and by their spatial circumferential continuity, from the prediverticular stage of diverticulosis where circular muscle hypertrophy forms peculiar cockscomb margins and transversal radiotransparent stripes in the intermarginal space (See Fig. 4 in Chapter 3).

The origin of these pseudoplicar formations can be postulated to be due to an abnormal motor activity of the muscularis mucosae. This muscle component of the mucosa, located below the lamina propria, ensures a motion which is independent of total colon motility, with the aim of favoring the release of secretions by intramural glands into the lumen. Hence, the finding of pseudoplicae is often associated to some level of local hypersecretion (See Fig. 4B).

On this basis, a retrospective review of the DCBE findings in patients whose final diagnosis was IBS was considered important, with special reference to the frequency of each sign.

In 1992 and 1993 in San Martino Hospital, out of 733 outpatients undergoing DCBE with negative reports for organic disease of the colon, at the end of all examinations 183 (82 males, 101 females) were

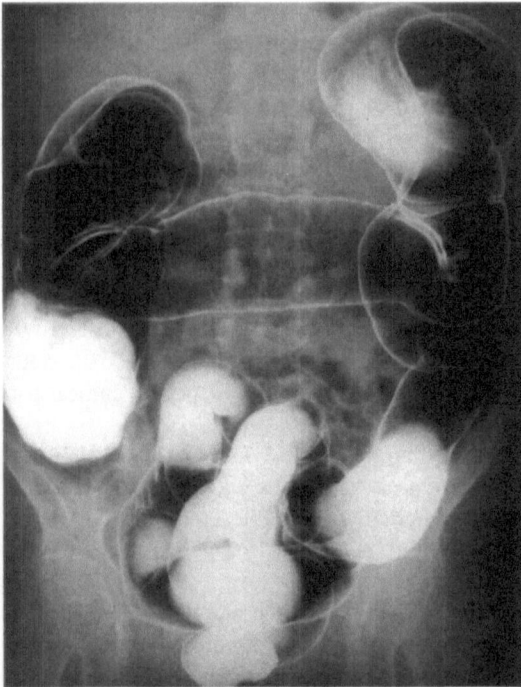

Fig. 1. IBS of the painful recurrent and periodic diarrhea type. Total absence of semilunar folds and haustral markings, which, according to Connell's law, is usually associated to diarrhea. A homogeneous increase in caliber of the colon can be observed

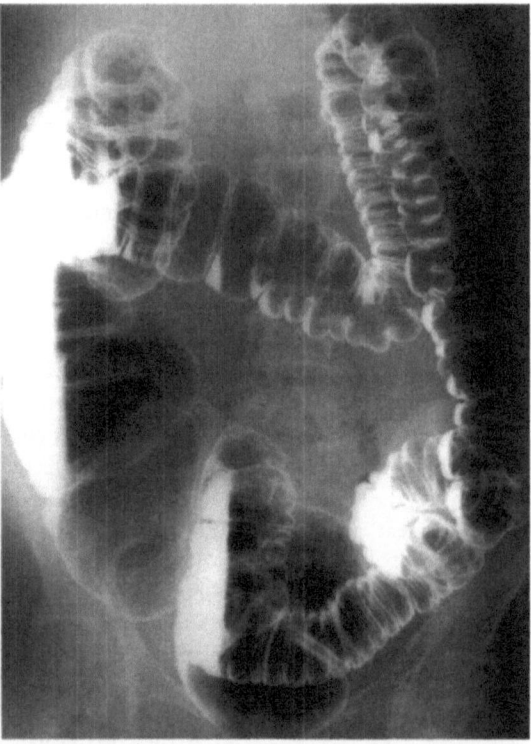

Fig. 2. IBS of the painful constipation type. Hypersegmentation of the colon which, according to Connell's law, is usually associated to constipation, affects the sigmoid (which generally has few haustrations), descending colon and left portion of the transverse colon. The normal appearance of the rectum, of the right portion of the transverse, and of a portion of the ascending colon and the cecum should be noted

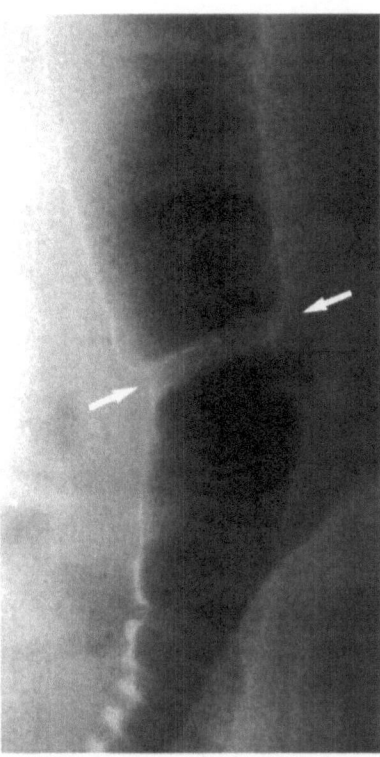

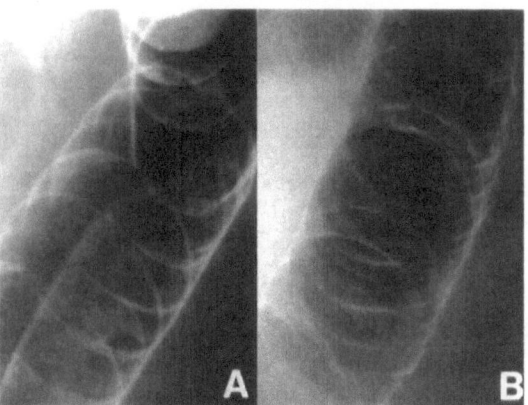

Fig. 4. Pseudoplicar formations in the mucosa surface. In (**A**), IBS of the abdominal pain type and varying bowel habit. Instead of the double "rail-track" appearance of semilunar folds, a single line can be observed with a more or less slanted arrangement to the major axis of the colon and stretching with a coil-shaped pattern along the major axis of the colon. Haustral segmentation is absent. Caliber reduction and contour alterations of the segment concerned are not appreciated. Abnormal motor activity of the muscularis mucosae was postulated. In (**B**), the picture is more or less similar to the previous one with some additional hypersecretion which breaks the thin coil-shaped barium line

Fig. 3. IBS of the recurrent abdominal pain type without alteration of bowel habit. Persistent narrowed annular segment at the site of Payr-Strauss sphincter (*arrows*)

recognized to be affected by IBS. During the same period, 65 in-patients (32 males, 33 females) underwent DCBE because of long lasting IBS. The age of males ranged from 21 to 64 years (with the highest incidence between 31 and 40 years), the age of females from 18 to 50 years (with the highest incidence between 21 and 30 years). Only 186 examinations could be recovered, 128 of which included all the radiographs of the standard sequence and therefore were suitable for a detailed analysis. DCBEs of 96 patients who had undergone the examination in the same period with negative report for organic disease of the colon but who were not diagnosed to be affected by IBS were used as controls.

The DCBE examination was always performed according to the Genoa technique, namely: pharmacological bowel preparation with sennosides, magnesium sulfate and hydration, without any cleansing enema; introduction of the barium suspension by gravity; on the spot hypotony induction of the colon with i.v. Buscopan injection just before air insufflation.

The distention and caliber of the various segments of the colon, the number and shape of haustral pouches, the presence of pseudosphincters, of pseudoplicae, the homogeneity of mucosal coating with particular reference to any local alterations due to hypersecretion, as well as any other findings were examined with the utmost attention. The results are summarized in Table 1.

Table 1 - Findings expressive of altered colonic motility in 128 IBS and 96 non-IBS patients

	IBS patients	non-IBS patients
Diffuse colonic distention	2	0
Diffuse colonic spasm	0	0
Hypersegmentation	9	0
Narrowed annular segments (Payr-Strauss sphincter)	4	0
Pseudoplicar formations	59	11
Local hypersecretion	5	1

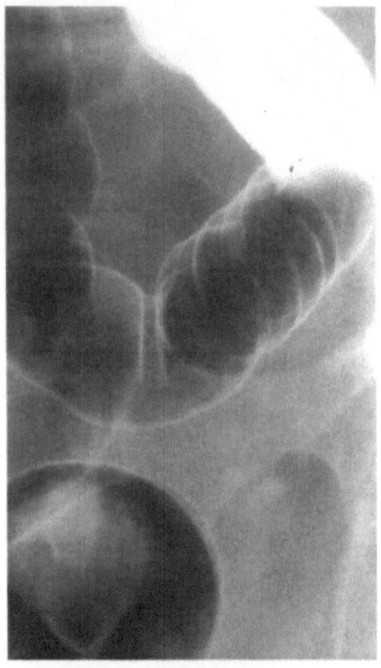

Fig. 5. Initial pseudoplicar formations. In this patient, a physician experiencing sudden work-related stress, the examination was induced by the onset of recurrent pain in the left iliac fossa. The coil-shaped pattern, well demonstrated in the anterior segment of the sigmoid, was the only sign. It had totally disappeared at subsequent follow-up, once the reasons for anxiety had gone

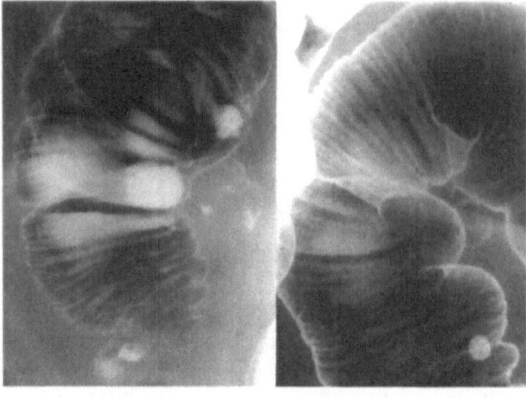

Fig. 6. Pseudoplicar formations. In the cecum and sigmoid the coil-shaped pattern is sometimes replaced by transversal furrows preventing full air distention of the segment concerned

Definite findings were observed in 61.7% of patients affected by IBS and in 12.5% of patients who, at the end of all the examinations, were diagnosed not to have IBS. In a global evaluation, this difference is highly significant (P<.01).

It is beyond discussion that none of the above described signs can be considered, *per se*, a specific pointer of IBS. Often they look like an exaggeration of findings which are not uncommon in normal subjects. Maybe they are only the expression of a colonic reaction to the maneuvers performed to implement the DCBE examination. Nevertheless, the far higher frequency by which they appear in IBS patients should be carefully considered.

Obviously, the elevated frequency is a direct demonstration of the altered colonic motility operating in this subpopulation of patients, such as to by-pass the inhibitory effect of hypotonic treatment. But what about the single patient? Although a diagnosis of IBS is evidently impossible on the basis of one or more of these signs, our opinion is that every sign should be meticulously indicated in the radiological report, putting between brackets a question mark on the possibility that IBS is round the corner. Which indeed is what we do as a matter of routine, without blame and with some praise. In fact, a good agreement between the above described findings and the final clinical assessment has been confirmed by the experience from daily practice at our department.

All the above would suggest that, when DCBE is performed with a soft technique aiming at minimizing any useless disturbance to colon functions - which is what seems to occur in the Genoa technique - it can give an important contribution to the study of IBS, *not only to exclude any organic pathology, but also to successfully identify certain functional motoric and secretory patterns.*

References

1. Thompson WG (1993) Irritable bowel syndrome: pathogenesis and management. Lancet 341:1569-1572

2. Jones R, Lydeard S (1992) Irritable bowel syndrome in the general population. BMJ 304:87-90

3. Almy TP (1957) What is the irritable colon? Am J Dig Dis 2:93-95

4. Kirsner JB, Palmer WL (1958) The irritable colon. Gastroenterology 34:491-501

5. Drossman DA, Powell DW, Sessions JT Jr (1977) The irritable bowel syndrome. Gastroenterology 73:811-822

6. Ruoff E (1973) Emotional factors in gastrointestinal illness. In: Lindner AE. The irritable colon syndrome, Ed. Amsterdam: Excerpta Medica

7. Manning AP, Thompson WG, Heaton KW et al (1978) Towards positive diagnosis of the irritable bowel. BMJ 2:653-654

8. Lumsden K, Chaudhary NA, Truelove SC (1963) The irritable colon syndrome. Clin Radiol 14:54-63

9. Teplick JG, Haskin ME (1976) Roentgenologic diagnosis. Philadelphia: Saunders, Vol II, PP. 914-915

10. Ritsema GH, Thijn CJP (1991) Painful irritable bowel syndrome and sigmoid contractions. Clin Radiol 43:113-116

11. Havia T, Manner R (1971) The irritable colon syndrome: A follow-up study with special reference to the development of diverticula. Acta Chir Scand 137:569-572

12. Kelvin MF, Gardiner R (1987) Clinical imaging of the colon and rectum. New York: Raven Press, PP 433-435

13. Cittadini G, Piccoli N (1980) The diagnosis of irritable colon is also a radiological problem? Proceedings of the International Meeting "Functional diseases of the colon". Genoa, June 1980

14. Rollandi GA, Sardanelli F, Mallarini G (1983) Irritable bowel syndrome and DCBE. In: Cheli R (ed.) The irritable colon to-day. Genoa: Scientific Meetings Menarini, pp 45-53

15. Templeton AW (1960) Colon sphincters simulating organic disease. Radiology 75:237-241

16. Janower ML (1964) X-ray seminar No. 39: Vanishing lesion of colon. JAMA 189:942-943

17. Gagliardi JA, Radvany MG, Kilkenny TE, Russo RD Jr (1994) Colonic sphincters revisited: simulators of organic disease. Hawai Med J 53:278-282

20 Radiology and surgical problems of the large bowel

Nicola Pandolfo

Today, in the diagnosis of large bowel diseases, several methods, often conducted by specialists of different sectors, are generally applied. Their technical features are constantly being improved and sometimes totally replaced by other newly designed techniques. If, on the one hand, this process favors an ever more accurate definition of the clinical picture, which is essential to establish better medical and surgical treatments, on the other hand, in order to achieve the best results, an adaptation to change is required, through adequate choices and a proper integration between the various types of examinations.

In addition, the selection of the diagnostic route is often significantly affected by the actual availability of specific professional skills and equipment in each center, as well as by personal preferences or simply by habit and more or less familiarity with each technique, with often controversial results. In the light of these remarks, we shall describe the approach to the major diseases of the colon-rectum-anus currently taken at the Department of Surgery of the University of Genoa, with particular reference to DCBE and the way this technique is applied.

Diverticular disease

A distinction must be made between uncomplicated *diverticulosis*, where symptomless diverticula, a frequent finding especially in the elderly, are detected incidentally, from *diverticulitis*, where symptomatic diverticuli are the reason for carrying out more or less thorough clinical examinations.

Recurrent and persistent disease, the onset of complications (hemorrhage; perforation; formation of fistulas in the bladder, in the small intestine loops, in the vagina; stenosis of the intestinal lumen; scarring from recurrent walled off perforations) and the impossibility to rule out cancer are indications for surgery, which affects less than 10% of patients [1].

DCBE is the first choice examination in preoperative evaluation, except in very active stages of the disease, when the risk of perforation contraindicates a barium enema. This examination gives valuable information on the disease evolution and to plan the exact extension of resection, to locate the site of diverticula, the actual length of the intestinal tract involved, presence of fistulas and stenoses. However, DCBE must be integrated with endoscopy in order to rule out, with reasonable certainty, the presence of a concurrent carcinoma [2] or, more rarely, of localized Crohn's disease. This is all the more important since, in case of diverticulitis, the intraoperative identification of a carcinoma may be very difficult. Crohn's disease was also observed to be associated in patients undergoing a second resection for diverticulitis [3].

Elective one-stage resection of the diseased segment is usually curative and associated with low risk for the patient. Emergency surgical treatment may be required in case of complications which have a high morbidity and mortality rate.

Idiopathic ulcerative colitis

Idiopathic ulcerative colitis (IUC) is an inflammatory disease of the rectum and colon, with lesions mainly confined to the mucosal layer, which may remain localized to the rectum alone (proctitis), the rectum and sigmoid (proctosigmoiditis) or involve the whole large bowel from the rectum to the cecum (full-blown proctocolitis). Though the small intestine remains unaffected, several inches of the terminal ileum are frequently involved due to abnormal feces reflux through the ileocecal valve (backwash ileitis). The external intestinal surface, which is not affected, is generally normal, except for a moderate reactive hyperemia. The intestine tends to be shortened in length and reduced in diameter, with loss of haustration and rigid walls as the result of a thickening of the muscularis mucosae and a tonic contraction of the muscle layers. In the most severe forms, and especially in fulminating toxic colitis, the muscle and serosa layers are also involved [4].

According to a currently common approach, in chronic forms with relative clinical quiescence endoscopy is the first choice examination [5]. It can be limited to the rectum, if pancolonoscopy is not feasible due to the patient's general conditions. DCBE is in any case indicated for the diagnosis as well as in order to establish the extent and progression of the disease and also as a reference point in the follow-up. In our experience, the two examinations have proved to be complementary in defining lesions and detecting the onset of a carcinoma in the colon or rectum, whose incidence is greatly increased in case of total colonic involvement or long-lasting disease.

An almost inactive and rigid contracted colon, with involvement of all its layers demonstrated by DCBE, is an indication for surgery as well as the suspicion of malignant changes during follow-up. In this latter case, as well as when looking for sites with severe dysplasia, endoscopy with targeted biopsies is an essential diagnostic complement. Total proctocolectomy with ileal pouch-anal anastomosis is the treatment of choice to permanently cure IUC [6]. Today, more limited resections with preservation of the rectum or ileostomy, poorly accepted by patients, as colectomy with ileostomy and mucous fistula, colectomy with ileo-rectal anastomosis, total proctocolectomy with continent ileostomy, are abandoned.

Total colectomy and ileostomy can be performed when urgent or emergency surgery is required, in the treatment of acute complications of the disease or when a patient is considered to be too ill to withstand a more extensive surgical procedure. The rectal stump is closed and an end ileostomy is constructed, the more extensive operation being implemented at a later date.

Emergency colectomy is indicated in the case of disease exacerbation, with fulminating acute colitis and impending toxic megacolon (which, when appearing as the initial symptom, may be induced by antidiarrheal medication, oppiates, belladonna alkaloids, by endoscopy and even DCBE) or in case of complications (perforation, massive bleeding, suspicion or demonstration of colonic cancer) [7].

In hyperacute forms, DCBE and endoscopy cannot be performed due to severe clinical conditions. Therefore, preoperative evaluation will be based on venous and arterial blood examinations and on a plain film of the abdomen to be repeated several times during the day. In any case, the patient is to be operated upon within 24 hours, that is to say before the onset of perforation which dramatically increases the mortality rate.

The plain film of the abdomen is taken to assess the degree of colon distention, detect the presence of any gas-fluid levels, of free gas in the peritoneal cavity, the absence of feces in the colon which is evidence of loss of one of the most important physiologic functions of this organ, as the container and transport means of feces. The degree of colon distention is a useful index to assess the severity of the disease; the transverse colon, which is initially 6-7 cm in diameter, progressively enlarges up and beyond 12 cm, which are considered to be an indicative sign of impending perforation [8].

In between the chronic, relatively quiescent, form of IUC and hyperacute forms, there are also active forms for which the DCBE examination can be employed rather safely in the diagnostic process. Personally, however, we would recommend some caution in prescribing this examination, also because the required information can be obtained with an SCBE performed at low pressure "by gravity", without any preliminary colon preparation [9].

Crohn's disease

Crohn's disease is a chronic granulomatous inflammatory disorder which may involve every part of the gastrointestinal tract. It almost constantly involves the terminal ileum, frequently the colon (in about 60% of cases), less commonly the rectum. Segments of diseased bowel are characteristically demarcated from adjacent apparently normal bowel (skip lesions). All layers of the intestinal wall are involved by the inflammatory process, with progressive evolution to stenosis and internal or external fistulas.

Colonoscopy with biopsy is considered to be the best diagnostic approach in the early stages of Crohn's disease [5]. In more than 50% of cases referred to us, the initial diagnosis was successfully made with a DCBE examination. In full blown stages, radiological investigations with DCBE, UGI study and enteroclysis are essential to detect all the segments involved as well as any signs of possible complications (sub-stenoses or stenoses of intestinal segments; perforations; presence of enteroenteric, or enterocutaneous fistulas). CT is also very important for these assessments. Recently, successful investigations have been conducted with In-111 labelled granulocytes [10].

Since surgical procedures do not have a demonstrable effect on the natural history of the disease, the rationale for operative treatment, undoubtedly affected by the very high recurrence rate, is based on the treatment of complications and prevention of intestinal carcinoma rather than to pursue the unrealistic goals of cure or reduction of recurrent disease [11]. Failure to respond to medical treatment, intestinal obstruction, intra-abdominal abscesses, internal and external fistulas, fulminating colitis and toxic megacolon, free perforations, massive bleeding, suspicion or demonstration of colonic cancer, severe extraintestinal manifestations (which seem to benefit from the removal of the most severely affected intestinal segments) are an indication for surgery.

Unlike IUC, total colectomies or proctocolectomies are performed only in exceptional cases. Segmental resections of the right colon are more frequent, with removal of the last ileal loop, as well as segmental resections of the small intestine or by-pass or strictureplasty procedures on stenotic portions. In principle, resections should be limited as much as possible, with the removal of the areas with perforations or fistulas, whereas stenotic portions should, as much as possible, be treated in a conservative way. All this, obviously, when the presence of a carcinoma can be excluded with certainty. Just like for IUC, the radiological suspicion of carcinoma must always be confirmed with endoscopy and biopsy.

Secondary irritable colon

Among the various organic diseases affecting the colon, there are several disorders (i.e. benign and malignant tumors, segmental non tumor-related stenoses and substenoses, secondary dolichocolon) whose early clinical manifestations are similar to those caused by functional colon motility disorders. This is justified by the fact that lesions caused by inflammation or tumor in the large bowel may sometimes initially provoke motility and secretory alterations of the colon. The symptoms and signs are those typical of the irritable colon syndrome: i.e. abdominal pain, myxorrhea, constipation, diarrhea and alteration of bowel habit (see Chapter 19). The underlying organic disease is bound to remain unknown for a long time if it is not promptly identified through a proper diagnostic route.

The DCBE examination is a better first choice investigation than colonoscopy, because it enables the identification of any organic lesion causing the clinical picture or, if there is none, it helps to identify valuable findings conducive to the motility and mucous secretion alterations typical of primary irritable colon [12].

Colon polyps

A polyp is any formation, irrespective of its histological characteristics, projecting from the intestinal mucosa surface into the lumen. It is possible to distinguish between *neoplastic polyps* (tubular adenoma, villous adenoma and tubulovillous adenoma), *hamartomatous polyps* (juvenile polyps, Peutz-Jeghers syndrome, Cronkhite-Canada syndrome), *inflammatory polyps* (inflammatory polyps and pseudopolyps, benign lymphoid polyps) and *hyperplastic polyps*.

Malignant degeneration of adenomas depends on the histologic type and size of polyps. Areas of invasive carcinoma are rarely found in adenomas less than 1 cm in diameter; however, malignant degeneration is more likely to occur with increase in volume over time [13]. On average, carcinomatous cells are present in 5% of tubular adenomas, in 40% of villous adenomas and 22% of tubulovillous adenomas [14].

Consequently, polypectomy can be both prophylactic and therapeutical [15]. For this reason, all cases detected with DCBE must also be examined by colonoscopy in order to remove pedunculated and sessile polyps. In our Department, 1-2 months after the removal of all polyps with endoscopy we generally perform a DCBE examination to check that all of them have actually been removed. This examination, with which the whole colon can be easily examined, is performed again during the follow-up. Thanks to the high sensitivity of DCBE, new polyps can be easily demonstrated and suspicions raised about any possible malignant degeneration.

The surgical removal of neoplastic polyps is indicated in the case of a large sized polyp or when clear signs of deep carcinomatous infiltration are found by the histological examination of the endoscopically removed polyps. Surgical options include a segmental resection of the colon in case of early stage lesions while, in case of more advanced lesions, options are the same as for carcinoma.

In the case of familial adenomatous polyposis, whose carcinomatous degeneration in the colon or rectum will almost always develop after 40 years of age, radical surgery with ileo-rectal or ileo-anal anastomosis before the patient reaches that age is the only efficient treatment.

Malignant tumors of the colon

Adenocarcinomas are by far the most frequent malignant tumors of the large bowel, mainly affecting patients in their seventh decade of life. Less common are carcinoids, lymphomas, sarcomas, squamous cells carcinomas, plasmacytomas.

Adenocarcinomas may remain asymptomatic for a long time and be discovered only after the onset of obstruction symptoms (acute in 10-15% of cases) or, more frequently, after bleeding. As already mentioned, sometimes atypical symptoms, similar to those complained in the irritable bowel syndrome, may be reported. In 80% of patients referred to our Department, the initial diagnosis was made by DCBE, while the diagnosis on the nature of the disease is always confirmed by colonoscopy and biopsy.

The indication for surgery is self-evident. *Right hemicolectomy* for ascending colon tumors, *resection of the transversal colon including one or both flexures* for transverse colon tumors, and *left hemicolectomy* for tumors involving the descending and sigmoid colon are the available options.

An accurate morphologic study of the whole colon with DCBE is required for surgical planning, in order to determine the macroscopic features of the primary lesion, synchronous concurrent lesions, if any, in other portions of the colon (3% of all cases), sentinel polyps (20% of cases) and to raise the suspicion of extension to contiguous organs (US, CT and sometimes MRI are specifically indicated for this finding, also for a more accurate planning of a possible extension of the area to be treated). Firm stenoses, even of several centimeters in length, and fistulization demonstrated by the DCBE examination have not proved to be predictive of unremovability of the tumoral mass and, in any case, they are not a contraindication to surgical exploration. Surgery may indeed feature also merely palliative, resective and non resective, operations or the removal of peritoneal or liver metastases.

Obviously enough, all the above evaluations cannot be done when an emergency operation is required for sudden complications such as obstructions, perforations or hemorrhage. When there are doubts on the nature of the obstruction, the enema with water-soluble iodinated contrast medium and CT can both be useful, with the aim of finding the site of the obstruction and acquiring more data on the likely nature, respectively.

Malignant tumors of the rectum

These tumors are not histologically different from those affecting the other parts of the large bowel. However, they present particular problems to the surgeon, not so much related to the likely extension to contiguous organs and structures, but mainly to anorectal continence preservation.

With mechanic staplers, even low, very-low anastomoses and even colo-anal canal-stomies 2-3 cm from the anal verge can be performed with sufficient safety. Since the neoplastic intramural downward spread and the lymphatic involvement are rather rare conditions, it was observed that a resection of just 1.5-2 cm distal to the tumor site would be adequate from an oncologic point of view, except for poorly differentiated, anaplastic or too bulky tumors [16,17]. Based on this rationale, abdominoperineal amputations according to Miles are less and less performed, without any significant impact on the incidence of complications and, above all, of tumor recurrence.

However, an accurate preoperative evaluation is required in this approach to define the tumor size, its distance from the anal verge, its histological features, tumor extension, if any, to contiguous structures, degree of sphincteric function [18]. For these evaluations aiming at a better surgical planning, rectoscopy, endorectal ultrasonography, CT and manometry are more suitable than DCBE, which, instead, will be used to define the site of the lesion, to identify fistulas, and to look for any other concurrent lesion in the colon.

References

1. Letwin ER (1982) Diverticulitis of the colon: Clinical review of acute presentations and management. Am J Surg 143:579-581
2. Schnyder P, Moss AA, Thoeni RF et al (1979) A double-blind study of radiologic accuracy in diverticulitis, diverticulosis, and carcinoma of the sigmoid colon. J Clin Gastroenterol 1:55-66
3. Berman IR, Corman ML, Coller JA et al (1979) Late onset Crohn's disease in patients with colonic diverticulitis. Dis Colon Rectum 22:524-529
4. Lanfranchi GA, Labò G (1982) Malattie del colon. In: Larizza P, Manuale di Medicina Interna. Padua: Piccin, Vol IV, p 542
5. Gordon PH, Nivatvongs S (1992) Principles and practice of surgery for the colon, rectum and anus. St Louis, Missouri: QMP
6. Becker MJ, Moody FG (1986) Ulcerative colitis. In: Sabiston DC (ed) Textbook of Surgery. Philadelphia: Saunders, pp 1011-1023
7. Goligher JC (1978) The Surgery of colitis - past, present and future. Ann R Coll Surg Engl 60:258-264
8. Kramer P, Wittenberg J (1981) Colonic gas distribution in toxic megacolon. Gastroenterology 80:433-437
9. Thomas BM (1979) The instant enema in inflammatory disease of the colon. Clin Radiol 30:165-173
10. Saverymuttu SH, Lavender JP, Hodgson HJF et al (1983) Assessment of disease activity in inflammatory bowel disease: a new approach using indium-111 granulocyte scan. BMJ 287:1751
11. Drucker WR Crohn's disease (Regional enteritis). In: Sabiston DC (ed) (1986) Textbook of Surgery. Philadelphia: Saunders, pp 914-928
12. Cittadini G, Piccoli N (Genoa, June 1980) The diagnosis of irritable colon is also a radiological problem? Proceedings of the International Meeting "Functional diseases of the colon"
13. Muto T, Bussey HJR, Morson BC (1975) The evolution of cancer of the colon and rectum. Cancer 36:2251-2270.
14. Morson BC (1974) The polyp-cancer sequence in the large bowel. Proc R. Soc Med 67:451-457
15. Gilbertsen VA (1974) Proctosigmoidoscopy and polypectomy in reducing the incidence of rectal cancer. Cancer 34:936-939
16. Williams NS (1984) The rationale for preservation of the anal sphincter in patients with low rectal cancer. Br J Surg 71:575-581
17. Kirwan WO, Drum J, Hogan JM et al (1988) Determining safe margin of resection in low anterior resection for rectal cancer. Br J Surg 75:720
18. Mattioli FP, Pandolfo N (1994) Esiti funzionali nelle resezioni del retto basso. Boll Soc It Chir 15:52-56

21 DCBE and colonoscopy

The *propagation of cross-sectional imaging techniques* and the *competition from endoscopy* are the two major factors contributing to the 29% decrease in barium enema studies observed in the United States between 1975 and 1986 [1], and confirmed in many other countries all over the world. US and CT have made it possible to study abdominal masses directly, instead of indirectly through dislocations induced on the various intestinal segments; colonoscopy has taken clients away from DCBE for its great diagnostic accuracy especially in the study of patients with gastrointestinal bleeding or polyps [2-4].

Though it can be easily understood why the advantages of colonoscopy over DCBE and SCBE may significantly vary when described by colonoscopists [5-18] or by radiologists [19-32], the extremely negative opinion expressed by some Authors on the results offered by barium enema studies cannot be easily explained [33,34]. Have factors leading to systematic errors, such as priority given to one technique over the other, or different experiences or involvement in either technique by the operators, affected the results? Did the comparison refer to a poor barium examination and a good colonoscopy?

Our opinion is that DCBE and colonoscopy are complementary and not competitive procedures. Consequently, the concept of "relative" diagnostic accuracy has no more meaning, while maximum results in "total" diagnostic accuracy can only be achieved through an interdisciplinary approach.

The main advantages in the colonoscopic approach are the high sensitivity of this technique which, rightly or wrongly, has become the final arbiter of the presence of colonic disease [35], and

the possibility to take a biopsy of every lesion and remove almost all adenomatous polyps. Preparation to colonoscopy is as demanding as the one required for DCBE. Sigmoidoscopy with a 35- or 60-cm endoscope is normally performed without any medical preparation; conversely, sedatives and amnestics are administered before colonoscopy with medium length endoscopes by which the transverse colon can be reached and before pancolonoscopy extending up to the cecum, since these examinations, for the majority of patients, are more painful than DCBE [36,37]. The cost of colonoscopy is about three times that of DCBE [38,39]. Hemorrhage and perforation occur in about 1:3600 and 1:600 examinations respectively, and the mortality rate is 1:5000 [40].

Recently, the potential fallibility of colonoscopy has become increasingly apparent [41-50]. Lesions of considerable size may go undetected by endoscopy even when performed by experienced endoscopists: flat nodular carpet lesions with minimal variation in the appearance of the lesion from adjacent normal mucosa are the majority [50]. But, generally, colonic lesions are missed by colonoscopy mostly due to failure to examine the right side of the colon. Approximately 25-45% of colonoscopies, in fact, are incomplete and significant portions of the colon may fail to be examined, particularly the right colon, thus introducing a potential for error which cannot be ignored [51-53].

The major advantages offered by DCBE are: fast performance, less involvement for the patient, demonstration of the whole colon and of the last ileal loop, its lower cost and the significantly lower perforation and mortality rates in the range of

1:10000 and 1:50000, respectively [54-56].

In general, colonoscopy is more sensitive than the barium enema in detecting polyps smaller than 5 mm; for polyps larger than 7 mm, they are both equally sensitive [11,44,57]; the barium enema seems to be slightly more sensitive in the detection of cancer [58,59] (but the relative sensitivity may change in general clinical practice [60]), extramucosal lesions and extrinsic masses impinging on the colon. It is also more accurate in the evaluation of diverticular disease [61].

The advantages reported in the literature from combining, with one single bowel preparation of the patient, sigmoidoscopy and DCBE as a one-stage procedure [62-67], and, in particular, the fact that the radiologist, who is no longer required to assess the left colon, is now free to concentrate on the cecum, the ascending colon and the transverse, are fictitious. The investigation, as performed, must be global and comprehensive and cannot be mutilated by "disregarding" a portion of the large bowel (more exactly the rectum, the sigmoid and the descending colon) which is always so well documented in the radiographic sequence.

It is commonly stated that diagnostic colonoscopies are particularly frequent:

- where DCBE implementation technique is poor, thus failing to achieve the level of approximation to real anatomic conditions which the technique is supposed to offer;
- the organization of the radiology unit does not allow to meet the often massive demand for DCBE in reasonable time;
- the reliability of the radiological reports is not worth the effort.

In the centers where none of the above limiting conditions applies, endoscopy is justified, as second choice procedure, mainly in the following situations:

1. despite negative DCBE results, the clinical suspicion of colonic disease remains;
2. radiological findings of doubtful interpretation need confirmation;
3. targeted biopsy;
4. real therapeutic treatment (for example endoscopic polypectomy).

The reasons behind this approach are straightforward. However, a few explanations should be given with reference to targeted biopsies.

The diagnosis of the presence, location, number and extension of protruding lesions is very accurate in DCBE. Conversely, the diagnosis of the nature (polyp? carcinoma?) is much more uncertain, also because the malignant degeneration of a polyp, which macroscopically looks benign, can often be confirmed only through histology. Radiological signs leading to suspect a degeneration (i.e. diameter greater than 2 cm; major axis parallel to the colonic mucosa surface; irregular surface; retracted attachment base; short and stumpy stalk) are sufficiently checked by the histological examination. Yet, their absence, unfortunately, does not mean that any lesion degeneration should be excluded.

Therefore, unlike inflammatory lesions (and IUC and Crohn's disease above all), for which an accurate diagnosis is generally possible based on the radiological findings alone, in the case of large bowel polyps, a final diagnosis can be based only on the histological findings. Therefore, endoscopy is essential, not to confirm the presence of the protruding lesion, but for its thorough nosographic definition which can be attained only through an accurate histological evaluation of biopsy specimens. The great advantage for the endoscopist is evident, since he/she is going to conduct the investigation in a targeted way in order to find an answer to a question already raised by the previous radiological examination under the useful guide of an already available display of the exact large bowel anatomy.

In our center, the end results of a biopsy or endoscopic polypectomy are generally checked by DCBE. As a rule, the minimum interval between endoscopy with biopsy and the barium enema examination is 2-3 days after superficial biopsies, and one week after deep biopsies or polypectomy [68-70].

The screening for occult colonic cancer is a different problem. With a fecal occult blood test, performed every year, and colonoscopy, performed every three or four years, the probability of death by colorectal cancer can be reduced slightly more than with DCBE performed with the same frequency, but at a much higher cost [71]: therefore, a barium enema involving the examination of the entire colon every 3 to 5 years, would seem to be the most cost-effective strategy [71,72].

To conclude, we agree with Ott, Gelfand and Ramquist [35] on the fact that the complementary roles of an accurately performed barium enema and colonoscopy should receive increasing emphasis. As noted by Dodd [73], it is a mistake to place colonoscopy and barium enema in competitive positions: the two methods ideally complement one another, and when the examinations are used in the proper sequence, they provide a cost-effective approach to the early detection and control of cancer of the large bowel. Margulis and Thoeni [74] also recognize the complementary nature of colonoscopy, unsurpassed for resolving diagnostic problems posed by the radiographic examinations: this examination, however, should not be performed as the primary or screening examination of the large bowel except in special circumstances such as acute colonic bleeding.

In his Annual oration 1989 "Bring out your barium", Simpkins [75] stated that "a critical review of the use of barium examinations of the gastrointestinal tract compared with endoscopy provides evidence of a valid role for barium studies in contemporary radiology. It is concluded that there is no clinical, scientific, or economic justification for the wholesale replacement of barium radiology by endoscopy".

Furthermore, Stevenson [76] noted that "there is a real fear that enthusiastic use of endoscopy which at first stimulated an improvement in barium radiology, may end by killing what is still a valuable and needed technique". A further reduction in the number of barium investigations could be detrimental for the actual training and skill development of radiology residents, leading to a vicious circle (poor technical execution, more frequent diagnostic mistakes, less frequent demand for this type of investigation). The proper solution has to be found in stimulating a better collaboration between the endoscopic and radiological units. Only through a serene evaluation can objective decisions be taken on the type of investigation method required exclusively in the patient's best interest. The whole issue has recently been discussed in Italy, also with reference to the new requirements arising from the advent of endoscopic ultrasonography [77].

References

1. Gelfand DW, Ott DJ, Chen YM (1987) Decreasing numbers of gastrointestinal studies: report of data from 69 radiologic practices. AJR 148:1133-1136
2. Reilly JC, Rusin LC, Theuerkauf FJ Jr (1982) Colonoscopy: its role in cancer of the colon and rectum. Dis Colon Rectum 25:532-538
3. Spiegel MK, Johannes RS, Hendrix TR (1984) Clinical decision analysis applied to patients with a positive fecal occult blood test. Gastrointest Endosc 30:145-146
4. Stroehlein JR, Goulston K, Hunt RH (1984) Diagnostic approach to evaluating the case of a positive fecal occult blood test. CA 34:148-157
5. Teague RH, Salmon PR, Read AE (1973) Fiberoptic examination of the colon: a review of 255 cases. Gut 14:139-142
6. Sugarbaker PH, Vineyard GC, Lewicki AM et al (1974) Colonoscopy in the management of diseases of the colon and rectum. Surg Gynecol Obstet 139:341-349
7. Loose HWC, Williams CB (1974) Barium enema versus colonoscopy. Proc R Soc Med 67:1033-1036
8. Williams CB, Hunt RH, Loose H et al (1974) Colonoscopy in the management of colon polyps. Br J Surg 61:673-682
9. Wolff WI, Shinya H, Geffen A et al (1975) Comparison of colonoscopy and the contrast enema in five hundred patients with colorectal disease. Am J Surg 129:181-186
10. Kronborg O, Ostergard A (1975) Evaluation of the barium-enema examination and colonoscopy in diagnosis of colonic cancer. Dis Colon Rectum 18:674-677
11. Williams CB, Macrae FA, Bartram CI (1982) A prospective study of diagnostic methods in adenoma follow-up. Endoscopy 14:74-78
12. Farrands PA, Vellacott KD, Amar SS et al (1983) Flexible fiberoptic sigmoidoscopy and double-contrast barium-enema examination in the identification of adenomas and carcinoma of the colon. Dis Colon Rectum 26:725-727
13. Kjaergard H, Nordkild P, Hennild V et al (1986) Follow-up study after colorectal polypectomy: the predictive value of a negative double-contrast barium enema. Scand J Gastroenterol 21:353-356
14. Durdey P, Weston PM, Williams NS (1987) Colonoscopy or barium enema as initial investigation of colonic disease. Lancet 2:549-551
15. Lindsay DC, Freeman JG, Cobden (1988) I et al Should colonoscopy be the first investigation for colonic disease? BMJ 296:167-169
16. Nelgut AI, Forde KA (1988) Screening colonoscopy: has the time come? Am J Gastroenterol 83:295-296
17. Warden MJ, Petrelli NJ, Herrera L et al (1988) Endoscopy versus double-contrast barium enema in the evaluation of patients with symptoms suggestive of colorectal carcinoma. Am J Surg 155:224-226
18. Irvine EJ, O'Connor J, Frost RA et al (1988) Prospective comparison of double contrast barium enema plus flexible sigmoidoscopy colonoscopy in rectal bleeding: Barium enema vs. colonoscopy in rectal bleeding. Gut 29:1188-1193
19. Laufer I, Mullens JE, Hamilton J (1976) Correlation of endoscopy and double-contrast radiography in the early stages of ulcerative and granulomatous colitis. Radiology 118:1-5
20. Thoeni RF, Margulis AR (1978) The state of radiographic technique in the examination of the colon: a survey. Radiology 127:317-323
21. Thoeni RF (1981 Double-contrast barium enema and colonoscopy: where do we stand? In: Margulis AR, Gooding CA (eds.) Diagnostic Radiology. San Francisco: UCSF

Extended Programs in Medical Education, pp 81-90

22. Evers K, Laufer I, Gordon RL et al (1981) Double-contrast enema examination for detection of rectal carcinoma. Radiology 140:635-639

23. Thoeni RF, Petras A (1982) Detection of rectal and rectosigmoid lesions by double-contrast barium enema and sigmoidoscopy: accuracy of technique and efficacy of standard overhead views. Radiology 142:59-62

24. Thoeni RF, Venbrux AC (1983) The value of colonoscopy and double-contrast barium-enema examination in the evaluation of patients with subacute and chronic lower intestinal bleeding. Radiology 146:603-607

25. Maurer HJ, Bieber M, Lange U (1985) Comments on the value of X-ray contrast examination of the colon (Germ). Roentgenbl 38:296-300

26. Jensen J, Kewenter J, Haglind E et al (1986) Diagnostic accuracy of double-contrast enema and rectosigmoidoscopy in connection with faecal occult blood testing for the detection of rectosigmoid neoplasms. Br J Surg 73: 961-964

27. Chen YM, Ott DJ, Gelfand DW et al (1988) Impact of the barium enema on patient management. Gastrointest Radiol 13:81-84

28. Gelfand DW (1988) Gastrointestinal radiology: A short history and predictions for the future. AJR 150:727-730

29. Jaramillo E, Slezak P (1992) Comparison between double-contrast barium enema and colonoscopy to investigate lower gastrointestinal bleeding. Gastrointest Radiol 17:81-83

30. MacCarty RL (1992) Colorectal cancer: The case for the barium enema. Mayo Clin Proc 67:253-257

31. Steine S, Stordahl A, Lunde OC et al (1993) Double-contrast barium enema versus colonoscopy in the diagnosis of neoplastic disorders: aspects of decision-making in general practice. Fam Pract 10:288-291

32. Brady AP, Stevenson GW, Stevenson I (1994) Colorectal cancer overlooked at barium enema examination and colonoscopy: a continuing perceptual problem. Radiology 192:373-378

33. Thorson AG, Christensen MA, Davis SJ (1986) The role of colonoscopy in the assessment of patients with colorectal cancer. Dis Colon Rectum 29:306-311

34. Norfleet RG, Ryan ME, Wyman JB et al (1991) Barium enema versus colonoscopy for patients with polyps found during flexible sigmoidoscopy. Gastrointest Endosc 37: 531-534

35. Ott DJ, Gelfand DW, Ramquist NA (1980) Causes of error in gastrointestinal radiology. II. Barium enema examination. Gastrointest Radiol 5:99-105

36. Van Ness MM, Chobianian SJ, Winters C et al (1987) A study of patient acceptance of double-contrast barium enema and colonoscopy: which procedure is preferred by patients? Arch Intern Med 147:2175-2176

37. Steine S (1994) Which hurts the most? A comparison of pain rating during double-contrast barium enema examination and colonoscopy. Radiology 191:99-101

38. Ott DJ, Gelfand DW, Chen YM et al (1985) Colonoscopy and the barium enema: A radiologic viewpoint. South Med J 78:1033-1035

39. Feczko PJ, Halpert RD (1986) Reassessing the role of radi-

ology in hemoccult screening. AJR 146:697-701

40. Habr-Gama A, Waye JD (1989) Complications and hazards of gastrointestinal endoscopy. World J Surg 13:193-201

41. Laufer I, Smith NCW, Mullens JE (1976) Radiological demonstration of colorectal polyps undetected by endoscopy. Gastroenterology 70:167-170

42. Leinicke JL, Dodds WJ, Hogan WJ et al (1977) A comparison of colonoscopy and roentgenography for detecting polypoid lesions of the colon. Gastrointest Radiol 2:125-128

43. Thoeni RF, Menuck L (1977) Comparison of barium enema and colonoscopy in detection of small colonic polyps. Radiology 124:631-635

44. Dodds WJ, Stewart EM, Hogan WJ (1977) Role of colonoscopy and roentgenology in the detection of polypoid colonic lesions. Am J Dig Dis 22:646-650

45. Miller RE, Lehman G (1978) Polypoid colonic lesions undetected by endoscopy. Radiology 129:295

46. Maruyama M (1978) Radiologic Diagnosis of Polyps and Carcinoma of the Large Bowel. Tokyo: Igaku-Shoin, pp 56-57

47. Fork FT (1981) Double contrast enema and colonoscopy in polyp detection. Gut 222:971-977

48. Thoeni RF, Petras A (1982) Double-contrast barium enema examination and endoscopy in the detection of polypoid lesions in the cecum and ascending colon. Radiology 144:257-262

49. Frager DH, Frager JD, Wolf EL et al (1987) Problems in the colonoscopic localization of tumors: continued values of the barium enema. Gastrointest Radiol 12:343-346

50. Glick SN, Teplick SK, Balfe DM et al (1989) Large colonic neoplasms missed by endoscopy. AJR 152:513-517

51. Alridge MC, Sim AJ (1986) Colonoscopy findings in symptomatic patients without X-ray evidence of colonic neoplasma. Lancet 2:833-834

52. Gelfand DW, Wu WC, Ott DJ (1979) The extent of successful colonoscopy: its implication for the radiologist. Gastrointest Radiol 4:75-78

53. Hagenthau P, Wagner HJ, Stinner B et al (1995) The value of double contrast colon imaging in inadequate coloscopic diagnosis. Radiologe 35:356-360

54. Masel H, Masel JP, Casey KV (1971) A survey of colon examination techniques in Australia and New Zealand with a review of complications. Australas Radiol 15:140-147

55. Gardiner H, Miller RE (1973) Barium peritonitis: a new therapeutic approach. Am J Surg 125:350-352

56. Han SY, Tishler JM (1982) Perforation of the colon above the peritoneal reflection during the barium-enema examination. Radiology 144:253-255

57. Waye J, Braunfield S (1982) Surveillance intervals after colonoscopic polipectomy. Endoscopy 14:79-81

58. Fork FT, Lindstrom C, Ekelund GR (1983) Reliability of routine double contrast examination of the large bowel: a prospective clinical study. Gastrointest Radiol 8:163-172

59. Beggs I, Thomas BM (1983) Diagnosis of carcinoma of the colon by barium enema. Clin Radiol 34:423-425

60. Rex DK, Rahmani EY, Haseman JH et al (1997) Relative sensitivity of colonoscopy and barium enema for detection

of colorectal cancer in clinical practice. Gastroenterology 112:17-23

61. Laufer I (See Whalen E) (1990) Colon Cancer: Diagnosis in an era of cost containement. ACR Conference, November 8, 1989. AJR 154:875-881

62. Saito Y, Szelac P, Rubio C (1989) The diagnostic value of combining flexible sigmoidoscopy and double-contrast barium enema as a one-stage procedure. Gastrointest Radiol 14:357-359

63. Hixson LJ, Sampliner RE, Chernin M et al (1989) Limitations of combined flexible sigmoidoscopy and double contrast barium enema in patients with rectal bleeding. Eur J Radiol 9:254-257

64. Gelfand DW, Ott DJ (1990) Limitations of combined flexible sigmoidoscopy and double-contrast barium enema in patients with rectal bleeding. Eur J Radiol 11:230-231

65. Hough DM, Malone DE, Rawlinson J et al (1994) Colon cancer detection: an algorithm using endoscopy and barium enema. Clin Radiol 49:170-175

66. Brewster NT, Grieve DC, Saunders JH (1994) Double-contrast barium enema and flexible sigmoidoscopy for routine colonic investigation. Br J Surg 81:445-447

67. Kewenter J, Brevinge H, Engaras B et al (1995) The yield of flexible sigmoidoscopy and double-contrast barium enema in the diagnosis of neoplasms in the large bowel in patients with a positive Hemoccult test. Endoscopy 27:159-163

68. Maglinte DDT, Strong RC, Strate RW et al (1982) Barium enema after colorectal biopsies: experimental data. AJR 139:693-697

69. Harned RK, Consigny PM, Cooper NB et al (1982) Barium enema examination following biopsy of the rectum or colon. Radiology 145:11-16

70. Bartram CI, Hall-Craggs MA (1987) Interventional colorectal endoscopic procedures: residual lesions on follow-up double-contrast barium enema study. Radiology 162:835-838

71. Eddy DM (1990) Screening for colorectal cancer. Ann Intern Med 113:373-384

72. Gelfand DW, Ott DJ (1991) The economic implications of radiologic screening for colonic cancer. AJR 156:939-943

73. Dodd GD (1992) The role of the barium enema in the detection of colonic neoplasms. Cancer 50(Suppl 5):1272-1276

74. Margulis AR, Thoeni RF (1988) The present status of the radiologic examination of the colon. Radiology 167:1-5

75. Simpkins KC. Annual Oration 1989: bring out your barium. J Can Assoc Radiol (1989) 40:5-11

76. Stevenson GW (1990) Radiology and endoscopy: commentary. Annual of Gastrointestinal Endoscopy pp 11-14

77. Cittadini G (1994) Radiologia gastrointestinale - Un crocevia pericoloso: ecoendoscopia o endoecografia? Il Radiologo 33(3):42-43

22 Enema, conflicts and perspectives: the psychological point of view

Novarino Rizzola

While, for a physician, speaking of the intestine means speaking of a specific organ with well known features and closely linked to the fate of another person, for the patient it is an inalienable portion of his/her own body with more uncertain boundaries; with its evil introjections, it can even undermine his/her residual physical capacity and his/her own safety. With a dual meaning, the intestine (or any other sick organ) may represent the oppressor but also the oppressed, it may be the area of a conflict which the patient would like to see limited and reduced, but could also involve his/her very Self for which a parallel and equally dramatic fate is feared.

With radiological exploration, the physician is already applying a brake and giving antidotes to the various opportunities the sick body has to worsen the situation even further, and to the uncertain definition deriving from verbal diagnoses whose connection with the disease is the only concrete meaning for the patient. The patient's imagination of his/her organs as a shapeless and unknown matter, where all his/her anxieties can be focused on, is restricted by radiological images. They help the patient to develop a sensorially accessible description of normally ignored internal parts, observing, with perspective realism, their current conditions, determining normal conditions and the evolution of any pathological process and, especially in cases of functional disorders supported by hypochondriac revision, thus setting limits to the psyche-soma-psyche vicious circle by which any already existing unbalance in the psychophysical personality as a whole would further deteriorate.

In addition to this ancillary psychological function, the radiologist, by moving "his own" defence barrier from the narrow relationship with radiography to that other "self in the world", which every patient potentially is, can address his/her technical activity and relationships in a more successful psychodynamic way. The various stages of the double-contrast barium enema examination of the colon raise several problems for both the patient and the physician: from the discomfort involved in the preparation phase, cleansing enemas (when performed) and the introduction of the barium suspension, to the proper examination, with all the specific psycho-radiological stress which is likely to develop, especially in case of functional pathologies or in the presence of diverticula or small polyps which are coupled to motor disorders of the bowels. On top of this, there is the opportunity for the patient to integrate the knowledge of his/her self and of his/her own body image, specially in cases of physical mutilation (colostomy), and there are also all the problems concerning the reporting and the relationship between the patient and the radiologist.

It is important to face this issue in all its practical aspects, since, by doing so, the radiologist will be able to conduct the examination while keeping in mind all the psychological features which may facilitate or hamper the presence, involvement and tolerance of the patient towards an examination which, if properly performed, may give precious functional information.

Personality and enemas

For every patient, the DCBE examination is more or less disturbing depending on how rigid is his/her character, how abundant his/her anal traits are, and also depending on his/her own sense of vulnerability. More specifically, previous experiences connected with earlier cleansing enemas interact with current circumstances, the type of approach, manual operations, the motivations and expectations of the radiological examination itself.

On the one side, the preparation, sometimes with the anguish provoked by excessively drastic methods, is a way to get rid of "ugly", "nasty", "infected" or "dirty" feces (adjectives by which the esthetic, moral, hygienic or conventional type of repression is immediately highlighted), thus leaving the patient cleaner and purer for the examination. However, the examination, as performed (the probe is introduced and subjugates the patient from the back, the lack of nobility of the parts under investigation), may lead to discomfort, signs of distance, poor involvement, annoyed detachment, and often to plead for a rapid relief from the neglected part, sometimes denying in advance any possible indulgence or pleasure, in closely intertwined real and allusive planes.

Though the evacuation pleasure is the spontaneously dominating feature in early childhood, there may already be cases of children who, on purpose, postpone, withhold their immediate satisfaction or inappropriately evacuate bit by bit, with an endurance sometimes close to masochism. Perhaps they sadistically deprive of this little gift - their feces - the other person, who is punished for his/her clumsy and often anxious demands, even before the beginning of the "pot struggle". This important issue is, however, less significant in the context we are discussing now.

The adult and mature individual, when faced by the medical prescription for enemas, knows, rather by transfer of old experiences than by current thinking, to be in an extreme situation and thus to be subject to the demands of the authority. For similar reasons, however, favorable and consenting attitudes are not often to be expected at the beginning. The immediate need is not so much the conscious realization of doing something for one's health, but rather, in the relationship's immediacy, the unconscious desire to meet the claims of the other, thus favoring a more tolerant attitude which, in the end, could even lead to avoiding the enema and related examinations.

Since many individuals yield into submission only when faced by a certain amount of pressure,

they often want to test the strength of such a "decision" through objections or continuous requests for further explanations. When the replies are weak and uncertain, a symbolic revenge for ancient contrasts is looked for, which will then come to nothing. Rarely does an envious impulse prevail, which aims at destroying the position and confidence of the physician.

The patients referred to the radiologist who has to perform the DCBE examination, have already been filtered by other physicians, therefore they are unlikely to rekindle the discussion. With their objections, they do not intend to avoid the performance of the prescribed examination, but rather want to make sure that it is actually and only to be done in this awful way and that there is no other formally more dignified mode (especially without enemas performed by strangers). Having been assured that the examination, for technical reasons, can only be done in this way, acceptance is the rule.

Some opposing attitudes may still remain, as sometimes is the case with young women, where tact and discretion are required. When those who have postponed or long opposed the DCBE examination finally accept to do it, it means that they are now sufficiently convinced and determined, perhaps by the simple addition of previous experiences or from the wearing down of their own resistance. With individuals who have a sufficiently solid and mature ego, who are content with a certain amount of realistic information on which they can carefully evaluate all the pros and cons, difficulties may be encountered only if the physician fails to give them sufficient consideration and useful elements for evaluation.

In general, those who really do not accept the examination do not even come to the radiologist except for children and adolescents who have to obey their parents. Sometimes they will take the opportunity to dramatically testify in front of the external authority, who may "still" be good or "already" contaminated, their subjugate condition and their desire to rebel, though they are themselves unable to find a constructive balance of power. If the examination is really essential, this should be explained clearly by talking alone with the young fellow and giving him/her sufficient time to compose himself/herself before the examination.

Paradoxically enough, indifferently obliging, often depressed people are those who are most likely to give up, to unexpectedly fail to keep their appointments. Their pervasive lack of trust for which sometimes they are disliked, is a sign that they do not expect any substantial help or improvement from the scheduled examination. They are suffering from a chronic, intensely yet generally felt malaise, which is only partially understood and accepted. Yet, they feel constantly increasing dissatisfaction and disappointment for their choices made in the past, and are reluctant to move in directions which, under a more comprehensive examination, would fail to effectively demonstrate their own abilities with sufficient safety.

Failing to come to the appointment is also an extreme, mostly unconscious way, to have the others look for you, thus confirming your value (and enjoying the care other people are demonstrating to you or the power of your own painful refusal). However, despite its obvious practical benefits, this does not occur often and, if it does, it is accompanied by criticism, thus further confirming that you are powerless and have remained outside the fight, rather than above it. A stiffening in one's still remaining features of superiority or some degree of depression are the logical and natural consequence of all the disappointments deriving from excessively absolutist, harsh and fundamentally narcissistic beliefs. Also they are the evidence of being unable to act and live even at a simple trivial level after having unsuccessfully waited for a messianic help. The individual is left alone without sure values, with thousands of possibilities in front of him/her and none of them credible, with a huge vacuum of pleasant object-relations. Even the external image of a more or less self-sufficient maturity may condition him/her against confiding in others on what really counts, thus perpetuating his/her isolation. With this type of person, in addition to constant attention and care, a revision of experiences and dominating values, of existential issues and the analysis of emotional rigidity is required, for which the contribution from a specialist may be needed.

Functional disorders of the large bowel

Large bowel irritability is such a common finding and its psychogenic origin so frequently demonstrated, that "irritable colon" becomes synonym for psychical, manifest or latent, conflicts. Even when an organic disorder is demonstrated, in which case concurrent and sometimes predisposing motor disorders are easily neglected - as if "psychogenic" were a convenient adjective equal to "essential" or "cryptogenetic" - the symptoms generally become more conspicuous or are even determined by a functional disorder of the colon, thus favoring an otherwise unthinkable organic diagnosis.

This is the case of people who, after a serious distress or grief over the death of a loved person, show a dyskinetic, improperly called "colic", symptomatology which, after investigations, results in the discovery of diverticula, polyps, if not even cancer, which otherwise would have gone undetected for a long time. Therefore, symptoms indicating an irritable colon syndrome, which could well hide an organic disease, should not be underestimated. At the same time, also organic aspects, the offsprings or even the relatives of a functional disorder which can affect their evolution in a mild or even severe way, should not be overlooked. An emotional component accompanies all colon disorders with a wide range of individual reactions in colon response to emotional stress [1].

Therefore, the presence of energetically contracted or segmented intestinal portions must be carefully reported and, when possible, connected with stress or with specific emotional factors (such as psychoradiological stimulation). The same applies to the hypo-segmented colon (which is a predisposing condition to diarrheal type irritable colon) especially where even minor movements are reported under emotional stimulation. In a poorly resistant and segmented environment, these movements are likely to enhance a fast progression of intestinal content, which in turn stimulates the remaining portions of the descending colon, with a rapid worsening of malaise.

The DCBE examination is suitable to make these comparisons, because of scarce internal stimulation caused by the low amount of barium suspension introduced and, above all, for the extremely detailed, almost perspective images obtained, with light and shade contrasts.

Reminding the physician that some organic alterations involving hypo- or hyper-segmentation may also be determined or "approached" by functional alterations which can be detected by the radiological examination and affected by emotional factors, as well as a good visual evidence and final reporting, can be helpful for the physician and the patient so that they will not stop at the first isolated malaise, but include it into a more complex objective analysis (involving local, general, personal, familial and social elements). This is the way to the discovery and the therapeutic analysis of a personal subjectivity with various degrees of distress, fantasies and painful conflicts. It is important to convince the patient not to unsuccessfully waste energies to limit improbable damage "directly" caused by modest lesions (i.e. isolated diverticula) but to focus, through the identification of a psychosomatic distress, on the involvement of the intestine "too" in a more widespread and alarming distress and on the psychoemotional, close or remote, causes of the patient's current illness.

The diarrheal type irritable colon, which some Authors suggest to be the substratum of the asymptomatic simple diverticulosis, includes well defined psychologic attitudes of abandonment, vain "fecal seduction" of the Other (feces as the ultimate present which, hopefully, will be welcome) and final desperation. Conversely, diverticula in spastic diverticulosis are not asymptomatic. This disease is thought to evolve from the spastic variety of the irritable colon syndrome, thus justifying the fact that pain and alterations of defecation precede the onset of diverticula [1]. A prompt and stressing reaction to disturbing events and thoughts is the psychological attitude, with an immediate tendency to resist difficult situations in a condition of concern and distrust rather than of real pessimism.

Something similar, but requiring greater care and medical and psychological counseling, applies to ulcerative colitis or granulomatous ileocolitis, which, though often preceded or accompanied by symptoms similar to those found in the irritable colon syndrome, present some differences in intraluminal pressure to be correlated to micro-circulation, lymphatic and humoral disorders of the intestinal wall. Both disorders are associated with specific and conflictual conditions (serious threat of separation or abandonment with alarming experiences of impotence in ulcerative colitis; significant stress factor, with precarious yet resolute maintenance, to a certain degree, of a favorable situation, in Crohn's disease), which are evident from the patient's history.

In the case of hyperplastic or adenomatous polyps, variations on an emotional basis of colonic motility (which may even be increased by the very disclosure of the disease) are likely to turn these disorders into excessively troublesome pathologies. Therefore, the value of radiological findings which do not contribute to strengthening misleading or reductive defensive attitudes is once more confirmed, specially in those cases where the organic disease, no matter how severe, may hide and perpetuate existential and interpersonal problems which, though serious, have a completely different origin which cannot be canceled by mere denial.

Psychoradiological stimulation

A targeted investigation on major personal, family or social problems, on stress factors, worries or hypochondriac appeal can supply significant information on their likely effects at intestinal level, if these effects can actually be displayed in radiographic images or colonmetrographic plots. Personal investigations have demonstrated that a colonic reaction is more likely to be spurred by some questions asked to the patient than others [2,6].

In an experiment conducted on 32 preselected subjects all suffering from intestinal disorders [2,3] an apparently simple question like "Are you concerned about your health problems?" has spurred a motility index (MI) increase from a baseline value of 7 to 75.4. Less concerning questions like "Do you think you have difficulty breathing?" or "Do you have a good digestion?" have increased the MI up to 17.2 and 13.4, respectively. Therefore, it can be assumed that the more a concern is credible for the subject, the more its recalling, though simply implied, can lead to significant reactions at the level of the organ referred to, but not only to it. No matter if one is an imaginary invalid or simply a hypochondriac: in any case, this is likely to have a negative impact on the part under anxious observation, with subsequent "objectivization" of whatever disorder. Hence, disorders, no matter their origin, can be rather easily self-fuelled by a worried individual.

In an experiment on 35 male individuals [4], colonic irritability and intraluminal pressure increase have been recorded more frequently when asked questions concerning their job ("Does your job cause you problems?" - 31.4%), prospects and skills ("Do you think that things are going to improve also with your help?" - 28.6%), jealousy ("Are you jealous?" - 28.6%), irritability ("Do you get angry easily?" - 25.7%), desire to change and regret ("Would you like to go back in time and change your life?" - 25.7%). The issues resulting to be more significant and frequent among women were slightly different as demonstrated by an experiment conducted on 45 of them [2]: dependence ("Do you easily rely on the help from other people?" - 31.1%), faith ("Do you believe in God or something else?" - 24.4%), social relations ("Do you like people?" - 24.4%), children ("Do you like children?" - 24.4%). Intestinal irritability favored by a mental calculation has been frequent though not very intense (is "3 + 19 + 2 equal to 24?" - 40%).

When the patient's situation and related problems have been examined in a more conversational, supportive and empathic way through psychiatric counseling, dysfunctions were less marked. In a study conducted during the presentation of some Thematic Apperception Test (T.A.T.) tables and the creation of related stories, 7 out of 13 subjects with previous intraluminal pressure alterations showed a considerable overall improvement in intestinal functions [5].

Therefore, the radiologist has the opportunity, after a brief analysis of the patient's character, to ask the most suitable questions for psychoradiologic stimulation, and, while the patient is busy answering the questions (YES or NO), his/her bowel image will be obtained and compared with the patient's baseline image without stimulation [6]. The radiologist then, after having identified the presence of functional disorders either in the basal condition or after specific psychoradiologic stimulation, if capable and if there is a good relationship with the patient, can go on with the conversation trying to better understand the information already acquired and its related problems, somehow taking advantage of the temporary "omnipotence" acquired with the complex and various tools employed and the findings already available.

All this will in any case facilitate the beginning of a possible subsequent psychotherapy, a referral to the general practitioner, a better self-esteem and understanding on the part of the patient of his/her emotional environment. The patient, who has acquired a clearer picture and often put into perspective his/her somatic and relational ghosts, has now acquired greater enthusiasm and courage to establish a deep dialogue on repressed traits, memories and problems.

Body image integration

The bowels, for their lack of reference to reality, once they draw your attention, offer many elements on which you can fantasize. Since, unfortunately, they are not visible, the idea you get of them derives from indirect representations (pictures, animal guts, etc.) which are often rather schematic and are rarely a true representation of your own insides. This leaves you with a very vague if not wrong idea of them. Hence, there is no clear or rigid boundary line among the stomach, the intestine and the uterus, or any other internal organs, "as long as they stay inside" or unless they are reproduced outside in a probable and personalized way [7].

With radiography and more specifically with DCBE, patients can get the most evident and often best bowel description, which can help them to develop a better image of their own inner soma [6]. If the bowels are proved to be more or less healthy - and an accurate description by the radiologist will certainly help the patient to better understand the situation - this is at the same time reassuring, educational and positively counseling. Functional disorders or minor organic alterations stimulated or highlighted by an irritable colon, may also confirm the possibility of regaining normal intestinal functions once stress and psychoemotional conflicts affecting the intestine are reduced (through education and counseling). When the somatic disorder is linked with the psychic element, the latter becomes the center of attention, "speaking up" again, and finally being treated together with the tell-tale symptoms.

On the other hand, when faced with an exclusively organic non fatal disease, a short-term revision of the disease ensures against excessive pressure on the Ego which, otherwise, in the long run, could become weak, insecure and pessimistic. That is to say, it is important that experiences of impotence, suffering and end of well-being do not crystallize.

Colostomized patients have particularly uncertain ideas not only on how their intestine looked like, but also on what was actually removed and what was left inside. Therefore, they must be helped to reconstruct their body image. Many of them believe to have been damaged and impaired more than they have actually been. As long as the newly fitted portion proves to be healthy and similar to the natural upstream guts, it is considered as a foreign element, which is refused and less controllable. It has to be loved in order to be able to love oneself again, and the DC image is, no doubt, alluring.

The radiologist

The radiologist, though essential in the display and sometimes in the treatment even of parts located deep inside our body, and despite his/her crucial role in the diagnostic and therapeutic process, generally has a tenuous and superficial relationship with the patient. Though any competition with other specialists or with the general practitioner should be avoided, being the core figure for a better diagnosis and therapy definition without establishing more direct connections with the patient and the other physicians may be somehow frustrating and misleading.

The radiologist may react by developing scientific or technological interests, look for other sources of power, favor uncommitted relations, may tend to get isolated. However, despite some gratification, all this will certainly fail to promote any better involvement and participation. Apart from cultural and historical factors (marked individuality of the radiological specialty school, ancient misunderstanding and distrust mainly characterizing the time of pioneering radiology), there are many other aspects in the defense mechanisms and character of radiologists that have so far favored this situation, and some resistance to a more direct and protracted involvement. Sometimes, they may appear reluctant to show how much they care for and need the others, as if they were looking for such an involving intimacy to be practically unfeasible.

Searchers - if not actually of souls - of bodies revealed to them, almost ethereal, "insubstantial" bodies, apparently without secrets yet full of shadows, they end up being the somehow detached witnesses of other people's lives. Only by trying not to be too technical or secluded, can they avoid being just the observers of their own world, with the risk of sometimes hiding important things which they could have mentioned (and done) and which perhaps nobody else would ever be able to utter or resume.

Therefore, it is important for the radiologist, despite all his conflicts or individual distress, to find, on a case by case basis, his humane and scientific way of "being together", and become another "physician available to the patient" [8]. If understood in a dynamic way, any failure or misunderstanding will just be episodes in the road towards greater success and a better mutual understanding.

Wherever the psychic system has failed and the organism has started to think, all relational, intellectual and affective values must be recovered with particular care [9]. The diagnosis report must be done with the utmost care and directly explained to the patient for the very emotional and almost prophetic meaning it has in the eyes of the latter. This report can give the patient, or at least not prevent him from getting, more important help and open up new prospects. When preceded by a good case history and a careful interview, these reports may also somehow better interpret concerns and uncertainties that have not always been expressed since the beginning. Too brief or too long, cold or doubtful descriptions, while not helping the patient, can even diminish the importance of a meeting which, from a certain point of view, is prestigious. Conversely, through a more careful and direct relationship, individual capacities and forces can be marshaled, with a mutual deliverance of physician and patient.

Finally, it is always possible to start from the radiological profession and find a common working ground for both radiologists and psychiatrists through the creation of Balint Groups: here, experiences, decisions and opportunities with reference to daily practice can be shared. In this way, working habits and relations are carefully examined, and the importance of apparently insignificant observations, as well as their value in daily work, become apparent, thus making participants able to muster the courage to acknowledge one's shortcomings and failures [10]. This experience can be the beginning of progress at work and in one's private life.

By focusing on daily practice, different aspects of the medical profession and individual mentalities can be critically examined. The development of personal, otherwise fleeting or unconscious experiences and observations will therefore give a significant contribution to changes in one's behavior. By merely integrating apparently irrelevant skills with abilities which are relevant to a certain sector or to a certain time (often the only usable ones under normal conditions) it is possible to promote that type of knowledge - mostly looked for and only partially given - with which the individual is helped to become involved in a wider consciousness, while acquiring better clarity, intuition, creativity and communication skills [11].

References

1. Sodeman WA Jr, Watson DW The large intestine (1985) In: Sodeman WA Jr and Sodeman WA (eds), Pathologic Physiology - Mechanisms of Disease. Philadelphia: Saunders

2. Rizzola N (1977) Significatività di un questionario psicosomatico nelle disfunzioni intestinali e nelle loro registrazioni grafiche. Minerva Dietol Gastroenterol 23:359-364

3. Rizzola N, Del Puente G (1980) Preoccupazioni somatiche e loro effetti sul colon. Minerva Med 71:1047-1051

4. Rizzola N Bertoglio C, Castellaneta G et al (1978) Frequenza di alcuni aspetti psichici nelle colopatie. Minerva Psichiatr 19:183-187

5. Rizzola N (1979) Espressione viscerale di conflitti con presentazione di tavole del T.A.T. Riv Sperim Freniatr 103:966-985

6. Rizzola N (1980) Turbe delle funzioni di eliminazione e clismi a doppio contrasto nell'ottica psicoradiologica. Il Radiologo 19(1):65-69

7. Ròheim G. The gates of the dream. New York, International Universities Press, 1952

8. Garrone G (1974) Lo psichiatra e la preparazione psicologica dei medici. In: Luban-Plozza B, Antonelli F (eds). Introduzione ai Gruppi Balint. Roma: Il Pensiero Scientifico

9. Ferenczi S (1985) Journal Clinique. Paris: Payot

10. Balint E (1974) Un aspetto dei cambiamenti che si verificano nei medici dopo aver frequentato i gruppi Balint. In: Luban-Plozza B, Antonelli F (eds). Introduzione ai Gruppi Balint. Roma: Il Pensiero Scientifico

11. Rizzola N, Nanni L (1991) La grafologia tra intuizione, scienza e coscienza. Minerva Psichiatr 32:193-199

Subject index